6/2014

LIBRARY
LEWIS-CLARK STATE
LEWISTON

D0392271

WITHDRAWN

Global Health and International Relations

For John Wyn Owen

Global Health and International Relations

COLIN MCINNES AND KELLEY LEE

polity

Copyright © Colin McInnes & Kelley Lee 2012

The right of Colin McInnes and Kelley Lee to be identified as Author of this Work has been asserted in accordance with the UK Copyright, Designs and Patents Act 1988.

First published in 2012 by Polity Press
Reprinted 2014

Polity Press
65 Bridge Street
Cambridge CB2 1UR, UK

Polity Press
350 Main Street
Malden, MA 02148, USA

All rights reserved. Except for the quotation of short passages for the purpose of criticism and review, no part of this publication may be reproduced, stored in a retrieval system, or transmitted, in any form or by any means, electronic, mechanical, photocopying, recording or otherwise, without the prior permission of the publisher.

ISBN-13: 978-0-7456-4945-0
ISBN-13: 978-0-7456-4946-7(pb)

A catalogue record for this book is available from the British Library.

Typeset in 9.5 on 13 pt Swift Light
by Toppan Best-set Premedia Limited
Printed and bound in the USA by Edwards Brothers Malloy, Inc.

The publisher has used its best endeavours to ensure that the URLs for external websites referred to in this book are correct and active at the time of going to press. However, the publisher has no responsibility for the websites and can make no guarantee that a site will remain live or that the content is or will remain appropriate.

Every effort has been made to trace all copyright holders, but if any have been inadvertently overlooked the publisher will be pleased to include any necessary credits in any subsequent reprint or edition.

For further information on Polity, visit our website: www.politybooks.com

Short Contents

Acknowledgements

We began working together almost a decade ago when John Wyn Owen, then Secretary of The Nuffield Trust, brought together what seemed an eclectic mix of scholars, practitioners and policy makers to grapple with the challenge of strengthening national responses to global health challenges. John's influence on this newly emerging agenda and, in turn, on our work in scoping out its intellectual boundaries, has been profound. For his early foresight in recognizing the collision taking place between the two worlds of health and International Relations, and the opportunities he then provided for us to learn from each other, we would like to dedicate this book to him.

Our early attempts to map out the common terrain between health and foreign policy revealed a rich seam of possibilities for new theory and practice. This initial work led to several fruitful research collaborations, with each of us bringing to the table careers and experiences honed from two very different fields. For supporting these collaborations, we would like to warmly thank Alan Ingram, Adam Kamradt-Scott, Sonja Kittelsen, Simon Rushton and Owain Williams for discussing many of the ideas in this book with us and, in some cases, providing insightful comments on chapters. A draft of chapter 2 was initially presented as a Public Lecture at the University of Aberystwyth in celebration of the 90th anniversary of the founding of the first Department of International Politics. Colin McInnes would like to thank Toni Erskine for twisting his arm into doing this. Elements of this book were also presented in draft form at a variety of conferences, workshops and seminars during 2010 and 2011. We would like to thank the organizers of these and participants for allowing us the opportunity to develop our ideas and for providing feedback.

The race to the submission deadline for this manuscript could not have been reached without the administrative support of Rachel Owen and Ela Gohil. Thank you for keeping us on track.

And, of course, books are always an intrusion on the lives of authors' families who eventually learn to cope with the erratic lives of senior academics today. We thank our families – Sally and Emma McInnes, and Andrew, Jenny and Alex Gilmore – for their unstinting support.

The research leading to these results has received funding from the European Research Council under the European Community's Seventh Framework Programme – Ideas Grant 230489 GHG. All views expressed remain those of the authors.

List of Abbreviations

AMC	advanced market commitment
APOC	African Program for Onchocerciasis Control
ARVs	anti-retrovirals
ASCI	AIDS, Security and Conflict Initiative
BMGF	Bill and Melinda Gates Foundation
BRIC states	Brazil, Russia, India and China
BSE	bovine spongiform encephalopathy
BWC	Biological Weapons Convention
CAGR	compound annual growth rate
CBRN	chemical, biological, radio-nuclear terrorism
CDC	Department of Health and Public Services, Centers for Disease Control and Prevention (US)
CIA	Central Intelligence Agency
CMH	World Health Organisation Commission on Macroeconomics and Health
CSIH	Canadian Society for International Health
CSDH	WHO Commission on the Social Determinants of Health
CSOs	civil society organizations
CVD	Cardiovascular disease
DALYs	Disability-adjusted life years
DfID	Department for International Development (UK)
DCPP	Disease Control Priorities Project
DNDi	Drugs for Neglected Diseases Initiative
ECDC	European Centre for Disease Prevention and Control
EDR-TB	Extensive Drug-resistant tuberculosis
EIP	Evidence and Information for Policy (WHO cluster)
ERIDs	Emerging and Re-emerging Infectious Diseases
FBI	Federal Bureau of Investigation (USA)
FCO	Foreign and Commonwealth Office (UK)
FCTC	Framework Convention on Tobacco Control
FIND	Foundation for Innovative New Diagnostics
G8	Group of Eight (G7 group of advanced industrial democracies plus Russia)

G20	Group of 20 (major advanced and emerging economies)
GATT	General Agreement on Tariffs and Trade treaty
GDP	gross domestic product
GFATM	Global Fund to Fight HIV/AIDS, Tuberculosis and Malaria
GHD	global health diplomacy
GHG	global health governance
GHSI	Global Health Security Initiative
GISN	Global Influenza Virus Sharing Network
GOARN	Global Outbreak Alert and Response Network
GPA	Global Programme on AIDS
H1N1	Swine flu
H5N1	Avian influenza
HINARI	Health InterNetwork Access to Research Initiative Programme
HIV/AIDS	human immunodeficiency virus/acquired immunodeficiency syndrome
HMN	Health Metrics Network
HPA	Health Protection Agency (UK)
IAVI	International AIDS Vaccine Initiative
ICG	International Crisis Group
IFFIm	International Financing Facility for Immunization
IGWG	Intergovernmental Working Group
IHR(s)	International Health Regulations
IMF	International Monetary Fund
IHP+	International Health Partnership Plus
IPPR	Institute of Public Policy Research
IPE	international political economy
IPRs	intellectual property rights
IR	International Relations
ISA	International Studies Association
IUATLD	International Union against Tuberculosis and Lung Disease
JALI	Joint Action and Learning Initiative on National and Global Responsibilities for Health
LMICs	low and middle-income countries
MAP	World Bank Multi-country AIDS Programme
MCH	maternal and child health
MDGs	Millennium Development Goals
MDR-TB	Multi-drug-resistant tuberculosis
MEDCAPS	Medical Civic Action Programs
NCDs	Non-communicable Diseases
NGO	Nongovernmental organization

NIC	National Intelligence Council (US)
NHS	National Health Service (UK)
NPM	new public management
OECD	Organization for Economic Co-operation and Development
ODA	Overseas Development Adminstration (UK); Official Development Assistances (US, OECD)
OHA	Office of Health Affairs (USA)
PATH	Program for Appropriate Technology in Health
PDPs	Product Development Partnerships
PEPFAR	President's Emergency Plan for AIDS Relief
PHA	People's Health Assembly
PHEIC	public health emergencies of international concern
PIPF	Pandemic Influenza Preparedness Framework
PPPHW	Public–Private Partnership for Handwashing with Soap
R&D	research and development
RF	Rockefeller Foundation
SAPs	Structural Adjustment Programmes
SARS	Severe acute respiratory syndrome
SWAp	Sector-wide approach
TRIPS	Trade-Related Intellectual Property Rights
UNAIDS	United Nations Joint Programme on HIV/AIDS
UNDP	United Nations Development Programme
UNDPKO	United Nations Department of Peacekeeping Operations
UNFPA	United Nations Population Fund
UNGA	United Nations General Assembly
UNICEF	United Nations Children's Fund
vCJD	Variant Creutzfeldt-Jakob disease
WDR	World Development Report
WHA	World Health Assembly
WHO	World Health Organization
WMA	World Medical Association
WTO	World Trade Organization

List of Boxes, Tables and Figures

Introduction

Historically, health and International Relations have largely existed as separate academic fields and policy arenas. The study of health, concerned with the physical, mental and social state of an individual and population groups, most narrowly focuses on human biology – how the body works, how it breaks down and how it can be repaired. However, it is now accepted that there are diverse determinants of health which must be taken into account. Along with biology and genetic endowments, these include personal health practices, health services, income and social status, education, gender, cultural factors, employment and working conditions, and social and physical environments. As recognition has grown of the importance of the broad determinants of health, study and practice has evolved accordingly.

Similarly the academic discipline of International Relations was long dominated by concerns about war, peace and security among states, concerns mirrored by the foreign and security policy communities. This focus, to a large extent, reflected its formal establishment as an academic discipline in the wake of the First World War, and in attempts to understand how such wars could be prevented in future. Over the next century, however, this focus has broadened to address new actors, new issues and new ways of seeing the world, a broadening of perspective also seen in the foreign policy world.

Like two cities with sprawling suburbs expanding into greenbelt, it was perhaps only a matter of time before health and International Relations would find themselves in closer proximity. While previously an occasional emissary would link the two, today there is not only the rapid construction of roads to connect them, but their boundaries are beginning to spill over. Both, as multidisciplinary fields, continue to struggle with questions of identity, of what they are – and are not – concerned with. Both, in practice, also struggle with a world of ever greater complexity and interconnectedness. Two distinct fields have thus been brought together in the early twenty-first century by the development of shared concerns, of uncertain disciplinary boundaries,

1

and of a mutual need for more effective policies in a changed and changing world.

The main backdrop to this development, as for so many other fields of endeavour, has been globalization. Health issues which cross national jurisdictions are nothing new, and collective responses to them form the very foundations of the World Health Organization (WHO) and other types of international health cooperation. By the late twentieth century, however, the scale and intensity of crossborder health issues faced by countries became far greater than ever before. Moreover, for many health determinants and outcomes, territorial space was being rendered irrelevant – infectious disease outbreaks, cigarette smuggling, counterfeit medicines, advertising of junk food via the internet, and the changing distribution of disease vectors due to climate change all challenge traditional notions of national health policy. To what extent could health continue to be considered as largely a domestic policy concern? How was health being re-territorialized, requiring new understandings of changing geographies of health and disease, their determinants, and the polities needed to govern them? The era of 'global health' had arrived.

Alongside the need to reconfigure how we understand the geography of health has been the reigniting of longstanding debates about the relative importance of biological versus social factors, the nature of health inequities within and across countries, the criteria for allocating scarce health resources, and even the definition of what health actually means. In other words, the paradigmatic shift from *international* to *global* health has challenged the health community to reflect on the intellectual boundaries of the field. Much has been found wanting. Few within the health world understand how the global economy works, why specific trade measures are adopted, what factors shape a country's foreign policy, how to conduct diplomatic negotiations and, above all, how such things impact on human health. These considerations are the stock in trade of International Relations scholars.

Conversely, this intellectual, pragmatic and moral struggle by health researchers, policy makers and practitioners on the effects of globalization has coincided with equally vigorous reflections on the study and practice of International Relations since the end of the Cold War. These concern not only what the 'new world order' looks like, and should look like, but what this tells us about the nature of the international system. Questions revolve around the continued dominance of states in the system and how we define state sovereignty; the emergence of new transnational forces and actors; and correspondingly, what power is in a globalized world, who holds it, and how it is wielded and to what ends. The boundaries of what is termed 'international relations' are also in question.

Most accounts to date of this growing common ground between health and International Relations point to 'real world' developments linking the fields either directly or indirectly. These developments include infectious disease outbreaks such as severe acute respiratory syndrome (SARS) and pandemic influenza; the HIV/AIDS pandemic in sub-Saharan Africa with fears of its potential to undermine the political and economic stability of states and regions; the broadening sense of what constitutes security amid the possible use of pathogens by terrorists (bio-terrorism); the impact of international trade agreements on access to vital medicines especially in the developing world; the increasing mobility of health professionals and patients across state jurisdictions; and the panoply of both old and new public, private and civil society actors in health policy making whose allegiances and resources crisscross the globe. All of this has prompted a perceived need for a qualitative shift in the nature of international health cooperation, a search for something called global health governance (GHG), coinciding with more flexible understandings of International Relations after the 'bonfire of the certainties' following the end of the Cold War.

This account, or 'narrative', on how health and International Relations have come together is common to much of what has been written so far in both the academic and especially the policy world. The implication is that developments 'out there in the real world' have made these links possible, desirable, necessary or potentially worrying depending on the writer concerned. The theoretical underpinning of this book, however, is quite different. For us, there is nothing natural, evolutionary or inevitable about these links. Although we accept that there is a material world which exists independent of our understanding of it, and which can produce risks and hazards to us, the way we explain and understand that world does not exist independently of us. We impose meaning on the world. The world, in turn, is thus *made* by individuals and communities (academic and policy). This places us in a broad theoretical grouping known as social constructivists. Crucially, therefore, the links between health and International Relations are not simply a natural and inevitable development arising from what is happening in the 'real world'. Rather these links are made, or socially constructed, in such a way as to reflect the ideas, interests and relative power of individuals and communities. These communities are not simply states, governments or political actors, but can include other groups such as practitioners and academic disciplines, in this case, within the health and International Relations fields. Each brings their own way of seeing the world, their own sets of explanations and their own priorities to the object of study. Indeed the very nature of the object of study, what it involves and what is excluded, is determined by these understandings of the world.

This social constructivist approach, as a starting point, has an important implication for this book from the outset. For us, differences in understandings are not the result of poor data, weak method or inadequate explanation, but rather a product of varied communities holding different values and interests. These differences are not readily resolved by reference to evidence or 'facts' drawn from the material world, not least because there may be differences over what pieces of evidence are considered important and how they may be interpreted. Oftentimes, these differences cannot be resolved, and competing understandings remain. On other occasions, these differences may be obscured by the use of common, yet ill-defined, terminology such as 'security' or 'globalization'. But when differences are resolved, they reflect the power and priorities of a particular community, including the power of ideas, rather than an independent understanding based on objective observation of the material world. The intersection between global health and International Relations is, in a word, political. Crucially, however, and an important contribution this book seeks to make, is the idea that these differences are not constructed by the simple binary divide of 'health versus International Relations'. Although on some occasions the different interests of the two communities may produce competing visions of the world, such a divide obscures the often contested nature of both health and International Relations, both as academic disciplines and as policy arenas. Indeed interests and perspectives (or what we describe as 'frames' in chapter 1) may be shared by elements of both communities but contested within each.

The aim of this book is to illuminate the social construction of the links between health and International Relations, premised on a shared focus on 'global health'. The numerous initiatives on global health that have sprung up over the past decade embrace the academic, policy and practitioner communities across both fields. Indeed, global health has become a major growth industry within higher education institutions (including a doubling of US undergraduate and graduate enrolments between 2006 and 2009), philanthropies, nongovernmental organizations (NGOs), consultancy firms, government departments and well-meaning celebrities (Wolinsky 2007; Macfarlane et al. 2008; Lederman 2009). Amid this enthusiasm, we begin by asking in chapter 1 what has been meant by global health, a question not as straightforward as it appears.

International Relations is by no means the only discipline to climb on board this juggernaut (Janes and Corbett 2009; Leach et al. 2010). International Relations, by virtue of its field of endeavour, however, seems perhaps the most obvious of the social sciences to offer substantive engagement with global health. Historically, health has never been confined by territorial geography, and great civilizations have been rocked, and even destroyed, by major disease outbreaks. In more recent times, the globalization of health determinants and outcomes suggests a close and natural synergy between the two fields. It is thus even puzzling that the two fields have remained so distinct for so long, and indeed, important to understand why, and on what terms, this estrangement appears to be being overcome. Why are bridges now being built between the two domains and what is the nature of these connections? This is the focus of the second chapter, which explores how and why International Relations has begun to engage with selected health issues.

The next four chapters of the book survey the common ground between health and International Relations, not to provide answers to major policy and scholarly questions such as 'what is global health security?' or 'how should global health governance be organized?', but rather, the purpose of these chapters is to understand and explain these agendas, the links between health and foreign policy, the global political economy, global health governance and security, in terms of their social construction. Our goal is to probe the intellectual parameters of this new field and the practical actions deemed appropriate to pursue in its name. How can we more fully explain the goals being pursued, the resources being deployed, the values being declared, and the curriculum being taught in the name of global health? We reflect on the nature of this emerging field – what Sara Davies has termed the 'global politics of health' (Davies 2010) – not simply in an attempt to identify what the field is or should be, but to ask why it is what it is. In this way, we seek to encourage more critical reflection, both in theory and practice, on the global health enterprise than it has received to date.

CHAPTER ONE

What is Global Health?

There is something ubiquitous about the term 'global health'.[1] In a little over a decade, it has come into common usage not only within scholarly circles, but as part of key policy debates about how health care services should be financed and delivered. Health cooperation is now no longer described as merely 'international' but 'global', as the scope for national responses to address a growing number of health issues (especially those with crossborder implications) is seen to have diminished in the face of globalization. Global health, in other words, has arisen in response to 'real world' developments that have led to the closer integration worldwide of the determinants and outcomes of human health.

At the same time, however, the use of the term global health can be understood, not only as a reflection of a profound shift in the ingredients that influence health policy, but as a concept that has contributed to that shift. In the creation and use of the term 'global health', a multiplicity of trends have been given a shared meaning which encourages us to see the world differently. Statements such as 'health is global' (Department of Health 2008a), therefore, are not simply a reflection of an external reality, but a rallying call to reinterpret how we understand health in a particular way. Health as global, in this sense, is normative in its framing or social construction of the subject.

This chapter explores these ideas in three main sections. The first identifies the orthodox explanation for global health as a product of, and response to, new trends, notably globalization and its impacts on health. The second discusses the manner in which global health is subject to different meanings because it occupies contested terrain. The final section argues that the manner in which we use the term global health is not value-neutral, but promotes certain issues, interests and institutions over others.

The Emergence of Global Health

Global health has grabbed the imagination of the academic and policy communities, as well as the general public. Within the academic world, the volume of articles, journals, books and book series has proliferated over the past two decades. This has included support for increased accreditation and training on global health, backed by professional health bodies and associations (Hotez 2008; Hogan and Haines 2011: 317–18; Lee et al. 2011: 310–16). This has been matched, and arguably exceeded, by interest within the policy world. New institutional mechanisms, arrangements and initiatives have flourished, many explicitly 'global' in orientation such as the Global Fund to Fight HIV/AIDS, Tuberculosis and Malaria[2] and President Obama's Global Health Initiative.[3] Indeed global health issues have become *de rigueur* among the world's most powerful people, whether at the World Economic Forum, G8 summits or the Organization for Economic Co-operation and Development (OECD). Regional and multilateral development banks, led by the World Bank, and other non-health institutions, including the UN General Assembly, have also given unprecedented attention to global health. This interest has been backed by resources. Health has received the lion's share of increases in aid funding since the 1990s (see chapter 3). There has been a boom in global health philanthropy since the 1990s, led by the Bill and Melinda Gates Foundation (BMGF), and with substantial donations from Bloomberg, Open Society (Soros), Warren Buffett, Ted Turner, and the Skoll Global Threats Fund (Stuckler et al. 2011a). Further afield, in policy terms, global health has featured as a rising *issue* in foreign and security policy circles, and as an *instrument* in the soft/smart power toolkit. Finally, global health stories (most frequently in the form of acute infectious disease outbreaks) have become regular fodder in the mass media including news, current affairs and entertainment.[4] In some cases, these different worlds have come together, as in the examples of media funding by the BMGF including *The Health Show* (British Broadcasting Corporation) and *Be the Change, Save a Life* series (American Broadcasting Corporation), and *The Guardian* newspaper's global development website (Doughton and Heim 2011).

So why has this remarkable growth in interest in global health occurred? One explanation is that it is in response to real world change; that is, as the world has become more globalized, so too has health. Up until around the mid-1990s *international health* was the more commonly used term, although it too suffered from definitional variation. Broadly speaking, within the public health field, four 'delineations' are often made between national and international health:

- international health referred to health in countries where imperialist powers extended their military and commercial reach, and after the Second World War to former colonies (empire delineation),

- international health focused on 'tropical diseases', reflecting a geographical focus on the countries of the tropics which suffered from such diseases (geographical delineation);
- international health referred to the health status and needs of populations in developing countries (socioeconomic status delineation); or
- international health was used to refer to comparative analysis of national level health systems and problems (policy delineation).

All contrast with the strict use of the term 'international' in International Relations as meaning between countries or states. In the second edition of his *Textbook of International Health*, Paul Basch lists a wider range of topic areas to potentially include under the rubric of international health such as humanitarian responses to disasters and emergencies, the ethical aspects of research and practice in poor and marginalized populations, and the social and environmental consequences of human population growth. The list is a long one and his warning, that 'a subject that pretends to cover everything covers nothing, or at least nothing very well' (Basch 1999: 7) certainly appears apt.

The replacement of the term *international health* by *global health* from the mid-1990s appears to have been prompted for two reasons. First, the new term offered a political boost to long neglected public health problems, notably but not exclusively in developing countries (Garrett 1994). These problems were not necessarily new but were either worsening, or becoming more visible, as a result of globalization. Stark inequalities in health between rich and poor countries drew particular attention. To some extent, one can see this as a rebranding exercise, putting 'old wine into new bottles', to generate political leverage. Linking health in developing countries to new agendas, such as security, foreign policy, environment and development, helped boost the political profile of health development.

A second, and related, argument was the call for a paradigm shift in response to how human health is being affected in new ways by global interconnectedness (some of which are identified in box 1.1). The emergence of 'global health' was presented, in other words, either explicitly or implicitly as a natural response to changes in the material world. As stated in the US Institutes of Medicine influential 1997 report, *America's Vital Interest in Global Health*,

> The health needs of diverse countries are converging as the factors that affect health increasingly transcend national borders. Among those factors are the globalization of the economy, demographic change, and the rapidly rising costs of health care in all countries. In a world where nations and economies are

Box 1.1 How human health has been affected by global interconnectedness

Among the most common changes identified as requiring a shift of focus to the global are:

- new geographical distributions of disease vectors,
- the emergence of novel infections,
- increased drug resistance,
- changing epidemiological patterns of health and disease,
- innovations in global information and communication technologies that influence health,
- changing patterns of health-related human behaviour,
- the global restructuring of health-related industries, and
- innovations in institutional mechanisms for collective action on health.

> increasingly interdependent, ill health in any population affects all peoples, rich and poor. As global needs change, the responses of the international health agencies are also being critically re-examined – a process that will in turn have consequences for health policies worldwide. (Institute of Medicine 1997: 11)

The world had to work more closely together on health issues because of shared interests in doing so.

The most commonly cited intersection of interests between countries was the emergence of acute and severe infectious diseases which have the potential to reach epidemic or even pandemic proportions. Science journalist Laurie Garrett's book *The Coming Plague* was among the most alarming and, some would argue, the most alarmist, published during this period. She predicted that

> [t]he history of our time will be marked by recurrent eruptions of newly discovered diseases . . . epidemics of diseases migrating to new areas (for example, cholera in Latin America); diseases which become important through human technologies . . . ; and diseases which spring from insects and animals to humans, through manmade disruptions to local habitats.
>
> To some extent, each of these processes has been occurring throughout history. What is new, however, is the increased potential that at least some of these diseases will generate large-scale, even worldwide epidemics. (Garrett 1994: xv)

The World Health Organization (WHO) was no less concerned. Director-General Hiroshi Nakajima, in the introduction to the *World Health Report 1996* on the theme of infectious diseases, warned that the world stood

> on the brink of a global crisis in infectious diseases. No country is safe from them. No country can any longer afford to ignore their threat.

> The optimism of a relatively few years ago that many of these diseases could easily be brought under control has led to a fatal complacency among the international community . . . Infectious diseases are attacking us on multiple fronts. (WHO 1996: 1)

Undoubtedly, this preoccupation with acute and potentially epidemic infections was prompted by long-held and deep-seated public fears of, and simultaneous fascination with, plague and pestilence. Such diseases attract the morbidly curious, drawing one's eye like a serious road traffic accident that we cannot quite look away from. This public interest was reflected in the mass media, with evidence suggesting journalists did not simply report on news 'as it happened'. Rather, in many countries, where health stories are among the most reported in the mass media, what health issues are reported and how they are reported bear scrutiny. Foreman found that what the media perceives as the highest risk to human health contrasts sharply with what actually poses the greatest risk (Foreman 1994: 7–11). This is supported by a study by The King's Fund which found that the news agendas of the print and broadcast media are heavily skewed towards dramatic stories and health scares, rather than issues that statistically have a greater impact on health such as smoking, obesity, mental health and alcohol misuse:

> The news media tend to focus on stories about health services. Only rarely do they publish stories about public health – that is, measures to improve health, prevent illness or reduce health inequalities. Public health specialists find it infinitely more difficult to cultivate media interest in serious, proven health risks, such as smoking, alcohol and obesity, than in, for example, 'crisis' in the NHS. Meanwhile, unusual hazards such as the severe acute respiratory syndrome (SARS) virus, which posed relatively little danger, can occupy the headlines for weeks on end. (Harrabin et al. 2003: 1)

Media reports, in turn, shape public perceptions of risk and views about the relative importance of different health issues. Such preoccupations can skew priority setting by individuals about their own health behaviours, by health policy makers deciding the allocation of scarce resources, and by policy makers far beyond the health sector considering how health fits within national[5] and global policy agendas.

The Multiple Meanings of Global Health

Paradoxically perhaps, amid the frenetic growth of interest in global health, a clear and agreed definition of what the subject entails has remained elusive. What are its intellectual boundaries? Are there agreed norms to be achieved? What goals define its spheres of practice? What is and is not a global health issue? Amid the vast literature that has sprung up on global health, both 'health' and 'global' (and especially 'globalization') remain subject to competing understandings and definitions. In this context, it is therefore unsurprising that the term 'global health' has also been problematic and that, indeed, we should perhaps *expect* multiple definitions given the competing perspectives at stake. In relation to health, while there is general agreement that the traditional biomedical model of health, focused on the biological causes, prevention and cure of disease and disability, is too restrictive, WHO's definition of health as 'a state of complete physical, mental and social well-being and not merely the absence of disease or infirmity' (WHO 1946 amended 2006: 1), has also elicited criticism for being too encompassing. Embracing both the biological and social are various wellness and environmental models, which emphasize the whole person and individual adaptation to one's physical, social and other environments, respectively (Larson 1999).

Three examples of how the biomedical and social medicine models might lead to different data requirements and policies are H5N1 (avian influenza), HIV/AIDS and tobacco control (table 1.1). A biomedical approach to H5N1 would emphasize prevention through vaccines, ring-fencing outbreaks and minimizing the spread of infection through anti-viral drugs, social distancing and quarantine. In contrast, a social medicine model might focus on addressing the conditions which allow the disease to mutate and spread, such as the habitation of chickens and humans in close proximity, or the economic conditions which lead to the non-disclosure of a local outbreak. Similarly, the biomedical model of HIV/AIDS seeks to understand how the disease is transmitted, how the virus replicates within the human body, and what drug therapies or vaccines might be developed to slow or prevent the spread of the disease. A social medicine model, however, might examine why specific population groups are more vulnerable to HIV infection, why individuals seem to choose to practise behaviours leading to a high risk of HIV infection or what forms of stigmatization might be preventing equitable access to treatment. Finally, in relation to tobacco control, the biomedical model would seek to explain how nicotine acts on the brain's receptors and leads to addiction, what the causal pathways are between smoking and specific types of cancers and other diseases, and how nicotine replacement therapies act to ease the physiological craving for cigarettes. A social medicine approach seeks to understand how children are susceptible to the marketing strategies of tobacco companies, what might be the best strategies to dissuade young people

TABLE 1.1 Contrasting policy interventions by the biomedical and social medicine models

Global health problem	Biomedical model	Social medicine model
Pandemic influenza (H5N1)	Treatment by anti-viral drugs and prevention by development and implementation of vaccines	Compensation schemes to poultry farmers, regulation of animal husbandry practices, reform of production and distribution of anti-viral and vaccine supplies
HIV/AIDS	Development of anti-retroviral therapies, clinical guidelines to treat co-infections (e.g., tuberculosis and HIV/AIDS)	Strategies for reducing engagement in risky behaviours by vulnerable population groups, education to reduce social stigma
Tobacco control	Analysis of nicotine receptors in the brain, development of therapies that interfere with nicotine addiction	Restrictions on tobacco marketing, advertising and promotion; youth smoking prevention programmes

from beginning to smoke, and how stronger customs and excise controls might be introduced to tackle cigarette smuggling. While table 1.1 presents these different approaches as divergent policy paths, in practice, most public health policies seek to combine elements of both. What is important to understand in contrasting these two very different perspectives, however, is that different models of health not only prioritize different issues but can also rule some issues in and some out of discussion. The ability to do this can be recognized as a form of power – ideational power. This concerns the power of ideas to shape our understanding of the world, and the power to promote a sense of what is natural or commonsensical, such that, sometimes we are not even aware of the choices we are making.

A second challenge lies in defining what we mean by 'global', including different understandings of the term 'globalization'. There has been perhaps no other subject that has elicited as much debate in recent times, eliciting passionate discourse about what it means to be global, and the benefits and harms of becoming so. Global is a word that defines a generation – within a global village, we are global citizens encouraged to think locally but act globally about our impact on global climate change, our role as consumers within a global economy or as part of the audience for an increasingly global mass media. For International Relations scholars, grappling with the term 'global' lies at the very heart of the contemporary discipline. In its simplest sense, global refers to a sense of the world holistically as a single entity. The world's division into 193 sovereign states, therefore, is but one way of viewing planet Earth. There are now many other organizing principles that shape how the human species exists and impacts on the world. Global thus threatens to shift the very foundations of International Relations, from interstate relations to social relations that follow logics defined, for example, by economic production and supply chains, ethnicity, gender, interests or technologies, and not the political boundaries of states. The resultant debates have been prolonged, nuanced and, above all, prolific.

Globalization, or the process of becoming global, has elicited a corresponding degree of reflection and debate within International Relations. What precisely globalization is, how we can measure it and, most controversially, what the nature is of its effects on our lives, has been given much intellectual consideration. Consequently, the literature is vast and ever growing, with no lack of excellent analyses available.[6] One particularly useful conceptualization, which serves us well in defining 'global health' more precisely, is offered by Jan Aart Scholte. He begins by arguing that

> [d]efinitions fundamentally shape descriptions, explanations, evaluations, prescriptions and actions. In other words, they affect our entire understanding of a problem. If a core definition is slippery, then the knowledge built upon it is likely to be similarly loose and, in turn, the policies constructed on the basis of that knowledge can very well be misguided. Hence definition is more than an academic and lexicographical issue. (Scholte 2000: 42)

Most definitions of globalization used in the health field are indeed 'slippery', serving to confuse at best, and obscure material interests at worst. Seeking to be rigorous in one's definition, about the distinct nature of globalization, is therefore considered by some an essential starting point. Scholte achieves this by identifying what he calls four redundant concepts of globalization:

(a) internationalization – increases of interaction and interdependence between people in different countries (i.e. crossborder exchanges);
(b) liberalization – a world without regulatory barriers to transfers of resources between countries;
(c) universalization – the spread of more people and cultural phenomena to all habitable corners of the world; and
(d) westernization – a process of homogenization resulting in the world becoming western, modern and, in particular, American.

He goes on to argue that none of these concepts are new and, most importantly, all are already distinct and widely used terms. All of these

Box 1.2 Examples of the use of redundant concepts of globalization in the global health literature

'the intensification of flows of people, goods, and services across borders.' (internationalization) *Globalization and Health* journal.[7]

'changes in cross-border flows reflect, and were preceded by, a considerable opening of economies, particularly in developing countries, through the lowering of trade barriers, removal of capital controls, and liberalization of foreign exchange restrictions.' (liberalization) (Woodward et al. 2001)

'a process of homogeneity producing a global culture sustaining the exchange and flow of goods and services, people, information, and knowledge worldwide' (universalization) (Cockerham and Cockerham 2010: 7)

'a thin disguise for a movement that attempts to integrate developing nations into the Western socio-economic and health care models.' (westernization) (Zimmet 2000)

redundant concepts of globalization can also be readily found in the global health literature (box 1.2).

Scholte identifies a fifth, and distinct, concept of globalization focused on 'deterritorialization' or the 'growth of 'supraterritorial' relations between people' (Scholte 2000: 46). This reconfiguration of social space, he writes,

> brings an end to what could be called 'territorialism', that is, a situation where social geography is entirely territorial. Although, as already stressed, territory still matters very much in our globalizing world, it no longer constitutes the whole of our geography . . . Geography ranks on par with culture, ecology, economy, politics and psychology as a core determinant of social life. (Scholte 2000: 46)

To date, scholarly and policy discussions of the shift from international to global health have been shaped by the above debates about the terms 'health' and 'global'. In other words, our understandings of global health are not derived from an objective examination of a world which exists independently of us, but by ideas which help us to explain the world. These ideas act as a road map telling us what to look out for, and what we can safely ignore. The problem is that these ideas are themselves contested, leading to multiple and competing understandings of, and visions for, global health (see box 1.3). Moreover, distinguishing between international and global has not always been straightforward, reflected in the manner in which the two terms have sometimes been used interchangeably. For example, the Canadian Society for International Health (CSIH) states:

> CSIH members share a common interest and commitment to global health, global health research, and international development. Our members include individuals

Box 1.3 The multiple meanings of global health

Multiple different meanings of global health exist, some emphasizing policies, some risks and others research. A number of popular examples are cited below. What they share is a sense that something has changed through globalization which 'transcends' more traditional 'national' heath where risks, policies and practices were largely dealt with by the state or by cooperation between states.

Health problems, issues and concerns that transcend national boundaries, and may best be addressed by cooperative actions. (Institute of Medicine 1997)

Global health is the health of populations in a global context and transcends the perspectives and concerns of individual nations. Health problems that transcend national borders or have a global political and economic impact are often empha-sized. It has been defined as 'the area of study, research and practice that places a priority on improving health and achieving equity in health for all people worldwide'. Thus, global health is about worldwide improvement of health, reduction of disparities, and protection against global threats that disregard national borders. The application of these principles to the domain of mental health is called Global Mental Health. (Wikipedia accessed 2010).

a field of research and practice that examines how factors of global, national, and subnational origins converge on a health issue, problem, policy, or outcome in an identified local social arena. This includes work that focuses on health inequities; the distribution of resources intended to produce health and well-being, including science and technology; social identities related to health and biology; the development and local consequences of global health policy promul-gated by national and international institutions; the organization of health ser-vices; and the relationship of anthropogenic transformations of the biosphere to health. We argue that the ultimate goal of much anthropological work in global health is to reduce global health inequities and contribute to the development of sustainable and salutogenic sociocultural, political, and economic systems. (Janes and Corbett 2011)

those health issues that transcend national boundaries and governments and call for actions on the global forces that determine the health of people. (Kickbusch and Lister 2006: 7)

an area for study, research, and practice that places a priority on improving health and achieving health equity for all people worldwide. (Koplan et al. 2009: 1993)

worldwide improvement of health, reduction of disparities, and protection against global threats that disregard national borders. (Macfarlane et al. 2008)

collaborative trans-national research and action for promoting health for all. (Beaglehole and Bonita 2010: 5142)

and organizations representing a broad spectrum of experience in various disciplines. Members contribute considerable time and energy to CSIH's many activities, programs and projects, and connect CSIH to other organizations in Canada and abroad. Through the engagement of its members and partners, CSIH endeavours to bring together various communities engaged in global health in order to promote a collective agenda.[8]

Moreover, others have seen 'global health' as little more than a strategic rebranding of international health. On changing McGill University's 'International Health Office' to a 'Global Health Program', its director Timothy Brewer pointed to substantive issues but also commented that 'Though names do not affect the smell of Romeo's rose, they have the power to conjure up images and associations when we hear them' (Brewer no date).

Despite the globalization of the term 'global health', what has therefore been far from universal is how global health is defined and understood. Is this lack of definitional clarity a problem? For some it is. Koplan and others, for example, argue that without an agreed definition of global health, it is difficult to agree on what global health is trying to achieve and how progress will be made and monitored (Koplan et al. 2009). Without a well understood, coherent research and policy agenda, multiple policies and initiatives emerge. At the very least, this is a sub-optimal use of resources; at worst, they pull in different directions or duplicate effort. The danger is that much of the public goodwill and substantial political commitment to improving global health, seen in the first decade of the new millennium, may dissipate as results fail to match expectations, a risk heightened by the harsher economic climate of the second decade of the millennium. Indeed, as early as 2007, Garrett observed that 'because the efforts this money is paying for are largely uncoordinated and directed mostly at specific high-profile diseases – rather than at public health in general – there is a grave danger that the current age of generosity could not only fall short of expectations but actually make things worse on the ground' (Garrett 2007: 1).

Beginning with the aim 'to shed light on the influence of global social norms on social behaviour and public policy, and to integrate into the analysis at times previously neglected normative variables' (Surel 2000), this book encourages a more reflective approach to global health theory and practice. From this perspective, the resistance to firm definition is a key part of the story to be told. The multiple meanings of global health arise from different, and often contested, normative frames which are discussed below. What is common across all of these different meanings attached to global health by health researchers, practitioners, and policy makers, in other words, is that they have normative underpinnings. In this context, the longstanding mutual neglect between health and International Relations, followed by the remarkable expansion of global health initiatives, tells us as much about the orthodoxy within these two fields as about changes in the 'real world'. Thus, despite substantial interest in the subject of global health, a single agreed definition is unlikely to emerge. Rather than seeking to reconcile these differences, there is a need to interrogate them more deeply and understand how they shape thinking and practice on global health and, more broadly, contemporary societies, public policy and world politics.

Competing Norms and the Framing of Global Health

The existence of competing norms, which privilege certain interests over others, is reflected in the anomalies of support for different global health issues. Why do some health issues receive more attention than others? Why is the health of some population groups deemed a higher priority than others? For example, diarrhoeal disease kills tens of thousands of infants and children each year in Africa but remains relatively neglected as a global health problem. Meanwhile, despite killing less than 1,000 people in total, SARS dominated the headlines in the first half of 2003 and much public health planning in its aftermath (Fleck 2003). This disparity between different health issues is seen clearly in funding allocation decisions. The massive increase in funding for HIV/AIDS over the past decade, including a six-fold increase in disbursements between 2002 and 2008 (Kates et al. 2011) has led to something of a backlash over 'AIDS exceptionalism'. Why has HIV/AIDS received so much of the limited available funding when other disease areas have received so much less? (Shiffman 2008). In general, infectious diseases have attracted the eye of old and new funders far more effectively than, for instance, road traffic accidents, chronic diseases and mental health (Shiffman 2006).

A number of explanations for the disparity between the global burden of disease and the allocation of resources have been advanced. Poor quality health information on the burden of disease suffered by specific population groups over time can certainly obscure, and even distort, policy decisions (Moon et al. 2010). The availability and affordability of effective interventions, or lack therefore, can also influence what disease areas receive funding, with donors choosing to do what is feasible rather than what is causing the highest levels of morbidity and mortality (Bloom et al. 2006). Misperceptions between the actual and perceived global disease burden by the public in high-income states may explain donor spending behaviour (Seigel et al. 2011). Alternatively, variation may be accounted for by the pursuit of material interests in the form of the lobbying power of patient advocacy groups, large corporations, governments or individual global health agencies seeking to feather their own institutional nests. The slow progress until the late 1990s on global tobacco control, for example, can be attributed in part to the significant and strategic efforts by a powerful tobacco industry to undermine policy action worldwide (Ong and Glantz 2000).

This book argues that what can also play a critical role are how issues are normatively framed, and the political purchase of these competing frames. Over the past decade, global health issues have been framed in a number of different ways dominated by five frames (see box 1.4). Each of these frames, based on a set of norms, privileges certain ideas, interests and institutions. In other words, each has particular answers to the questions of who and what is important in global health, and why. For example, framing health as a security issue would lead to the prioritiza-

Box 1.4 Competing frames in global health

Five dominant frames can be seen as key to the manner in which global health has been constructed in competing ways. These frames are not always self-contained but may spill over one into another, making clear distinctions sometimes problematic. Moreover, many of these frames are internally contested, with competing theories, methodologies and approaches. Nevertheless there is sufficient commonality within each frame to make them coherent, while the differences between frames render them more than heuristic devices useful for analytical purposes but rather a means of constructing issues in such a way as to suggest particular pathways of response.

1. Evidence-based medicine (EBM)

This frame encourages and reinforces positivist, rationalist ways of reasoning. It actively promotes the use of statistics, elevating this form of enquiry above all others. Decisions should be based on the best available scientific evidence using epidemiological and biostatistical ways of thinking. Use of this frame is often identifiable by the tendency to refer to 'evidence' to support decision making.

2. Human rights

This frame is based on the idea that public health policies should be based on the principles of dignity and respect for the individual. Programmes and practices should not violate human rights obligations concerning the avoidance of coercion and discrimination (including access to health care) and the promotion of transparency and community involvement. Links are often made to various international declarations on human rights.

3. Economism
This frame is based on assumptions that demand for health is inelastic (if you are ill, your demand for treatment does not vary with your income or the price of the treatment), and that the resources that can be devoted to health are scarce. The frame therefore lends itself to arguments about efficiency, choice and competitiveness in the distribution of scarce resources. Economics may also be used to demonstrate the value of health interventions in promoting economic growth, which in turn feeds back to increased resources for health or improved living standards which reduce health vulnerabilities.

4. Security
The underlying logic common to all forms of security is that of threat and defence. Health is framed as a security issue when it is presented as a threat to someone or something, and as something against which defensive measures (either in the form of prevention or response) must be taken.

5. Development
This frame is based on the idea that policies and practices should improve conditions in the 'Third World' where the 'First World' becomes something of a benchmark for measurement. Its central idea has traditionally been that of a binary divide in the international system between the 'haves' and 'have-nots' (usually expressed in economic terms) and the responsibilities of the latter to assist the former. Development as a frame, however, has so far proven itself to be notoriously difficult to grasp, largely as a result of how it overlaps with the other frames and adapts them within it.

Source: The authors thank Adam Kamradt-Scott, David Reubi, Simon Rushton, Owain Williams and Marie Woodling for these understandings.

tion of worldwide pandemic influenza preparedness over tackling infant diarrhoeal disease in the developing world. This is because the former, using a security lens, is seen as a threat to the core functioning of the state, while the latter does not. Correspondingly, applying the economism frame may lead to a greater focus on the health needs of population groups deemed the most economically productive in society (namely adults), and less priority given to the young and elderly. The human rights frame may lead to increased attention to the health needs of the poor and disadvantaged, especially in the developing world, including equity of access to health care and essential medicines, issues that would receive limited attention from a security frame. The development frame, in contrast, with its concern for poverty alleviation, might lead to a focus on endemic diseases in Africa rather than the risk of outbreak events (such as SARS and swine flu) spreading to the developed world. Finally, a biomedical frame would support the development and application of effective medical interventions that target specific diseases, and are delivered in health care settings, as identified by evidence-based approaches to policy making.

Of course, concerns about global health are not solely fuelled by cognitive frames but combine with changes in the material world. The historical relationship between patterns of health and disease, and the structure and composition of human societies, has been an intimate one. The globalizing world encountered by epidemiologists in the early twenty-first century is undoubtedly distinct, for example, from the slums of the industrializing mid-nineteenth century. Does this explain why there appears to be a larger number of new diseases emerging in recent decades than in previous times? Is it something about the material world, in the form of changing social relationships and, in particular, globalization, that explains new patterns of global health and disease? Haggett (2000), for example, identifies four changes that define the impacts of globalization on disease: (a) demographic growth of the host population; (b) the collapse of geographical space; (c) global land-use changes; and (d) global warming. What forces are driving their trajectory, how we understand the changes they are bringing about, and how we choose to respond to them all lead back to the importance of normative frames.

In this book, therefore, global health is located within a highly contested terrain of what Surel (2000) describes as competing cognitive and normative frames. He describes their role in policy making as the interplay of four key elements:

(1) *metaphysical principles* or 'world view' consisting of 'abstract precepts circumscribing what is possible in a given society, identifying and justifying the existence of differences between individuals and/or groups, and locating various social processes on a hierarchical scale';
(2) *specific principles* 'which allow the operationalization of values in one domain and/or particular policy and/or subsystem of public policy';
(3) *forms of action* that are deemed 'the most appropriate methods and means to achieve the defined values and objectives', leading to accepted practices and behaviours; and
(4) instruments or means by which accepted practices and behaviours are carried out such as institutional structures, administrative regulations and budgetary allocations.

Applied to global health, this framework helps to reveal lines of contestation, barriers to policy debate, limitations to practice, and relationships of dominance (see table 1.2). This approach opens up the study of global health as a social construct, framed in a variety of different ways, each with its own sets of interests, and with profound material consequences in terms of different pathways of response. While politics is often derided, as interfering or undermining forms of action and instruments of global health, most notably by the evidence-based medicine approach, this approach sees politics as central because cognitive and normative frames define global health and both promote and reflect different sets of interests and priorities. The most prominent of these frames to date – biomedicine, economism, security, development and human rights – are each characterized by a 'collective consciousness':

> Cognitive and normative frames allow actors to make sense of their worlds, and to locate themselves and develop in a given community, by defining the field for exchange, by allowing meaning to be conferred on social dynamics, and by determining the possibilities for action. They thereby contribute to the construction of individuals or groups as social actors in a particular field. (Surel 2000: 500)

In this respect, this book is a return to the roots of both fields. The systematic study of the relationship between society, disease and medicine, known as social medicine, began in the early nineteenth century (Anderson et al. 2005). It was during this period that Rudolph Virchow coined his famous observation that politics is medicine writ large (Ashton 2006). We argue that medicine, or more broadly health, must

TABLE 1.2 Examples of the cognitive and normative framing of global health

Elements	Examples
Metaphysical principles	• Health is a basic human right. • Health is a commodity subject to market supply and demand.
Specific principles	• ARVs should be provided free of charge to all who need them. • Donor agencies should involve local communities in setting their priorities. • Multinational corporations should ensure access to basic health care services for all employees.
Forms of action	• Use of economic incentives to promote healthy behaviours. • Encourage market to fill gaps in health care financing and provision. • Regulation of marketing and advertising of industry to protect children.
Instruments	• Levy on airline tickets by UNITAID to raise funds for ARVs. • Abstinence programme by PEPFAR. • Tax incentives to encourage R&D on malaria treatment and vaccines.

be equally understood as politics writ large. This book is about politics and medicine writ large together.

Conclusion

The coming together of political imperatives, not least in addressing global health inequalities, with rapid change in health determinants and outcomes, has produced a highly contested global health agenda. The construction of health as global, underpinned by the message 'we're all in it together', has led to an unprecedented focus on certain health issues perceived as posing risks to populations within and across countries. Jain (1991) argues that self-interest has been the primary driver, with global health 'rooted in the needs of nations, not in their desires or demands . . . This interdependence requires that nations work together, not out of altruism, not out of need to seek favors, not for reasons of goodwill, but essentially out of self interest.' Others see the growth of attention to global health since the late 1990s as rooted in a new kind of global consciousness, expressed through humanitarianism which transcends personal or national interests. There has been much talk of this global generation – those who 'want to make a difference' after decades of profligacy and consumerism (Panosian and Coates 2006). Global health recruits are described as the new Peace Corps, further inspired by the mega-giving of a new generation of philanthropists including Bill Gates, Michael Bloomberg, Ted Turner and other prominent individuals committed to 'making a difference' and 'giving back'. This commitment has been most pronounced perhaps in North America, but it is observable on university campuses across the world (Fauci 2007).

While it would seem churlish to criticize this new generation of activism, in a world seemingly in chronic short supply of such generosity of spirit, the need to better understand and where necessary, critically reflect on, global health theory and practice remains essential. Interrogating the normative basis of global health is an essential part of moving the field forward, both as a mature academic subject and as an endeavour to improve the health of millions worldwide. This first chapter has therefore set out to challenge the assumption that 'global health' is an unproblematic, rational response to exogenous developments in the real world. Instead, it suggests that global health is a contested field where different social constructions, expressed through normative frames, lead to different interpretations of what the field is, the goals to be achieved, and the policy pathways that should be pursued to achieve them.

CHAPTER TWO

Constructing a New Agenda: International Relations and Global Health

Why have health issues begun to regularly appear in books and journals on International Relations when, say ten years ago, this would have been a very rare sight? And why are health scholars, policy makers and practitioners increasingly interested in core aspects of international relations such as trade, diplomacy and foreign and security policy?[1,2] Health is traditionally seen as a largely domestic concern. Health policy is dominated by questions concerning how resources for health care are raised and spent, how to structure and organize health care services, what the balance should be between private and public provision, how to determine which health services and interventions are effective and affordable, and how to ensure the delivery of high-quality health care for individuals and populations. These questions, in turn, pertain to policy and practice within health care systems which, by and large, are traditionally confined within states. All this appears to be a long way from International Relations, with its historic focus on questions of war and peace, national security and 'power politics' (Wight 1979). Indeed, a standard textbook for the discipline by two US-based scholars, Charles W. Kegley and Eugene R. Wittkopf, explicitly contrasts the high politics of peace and security with the low politics of efforts to increase standards of living and improve quality of life. Health policy, from this perspective, would fall clearly in the latter category and thus be considered far removed from the 'high politics' concerns of International Relations (or in their terms, 'world politics'): 'In an unsafe world the search for national security has become synonymous with world politics' (Kegley and Wittkopf 1989: 351). This book is concerned not only with how this separation of spheres has changed, with health issues now featuring in both the study and practice of International Relations, but understanding why this is occurring and with what effect.

This chapter explicitly engages with the contemporary emergence of health issues within International Relations, and how health has come into the consciousness of the discipline's scholars and practitioners. Its purpose is not, however, to trace the evolution of this development by providing a historiography or intellectual history of this development. Rather, questions of a more critical nature are asked concerning what issues have become part of this new agenda and whose interests are served by this. Our position, therefore, is not one of rationalism – that the emergence of health issues is a response by the academic and policy community to exogenous developments in the 'real world'. Instead we adopt a more reflectivist position, seeing this development as a construction which serves some interests over others. As Robert Cox (1981: 128) famously argued, '[t]heory is always *for* someone and *for* some purpose'. In this vein, we wish to ask how the emergence of health onto the agenda of International Relations serves some over others and is for some purpose. The chapter begins by detailing why health was not considered a subject within International Relations for so long, despite longstanding international dimensions to health policy. It begins by engaging with traditional International Relations theory, especially the rationalist tradition exemplified by the two dominant theories of (neo-) realism and (neo-)liberalism.

Health and the Discipline
of International Relations

Although the academic discipline of International Relations in the early twenty-first century possesses a far greater degree of heterogeneity and pluralism than it ever has, in both what is studied and how it is studied, orthodox accounts remain organized around two distinct centres of gravity. The first concerns the subject matter. At the heart of orthodox accounts are relations between states (e.g., Waltz 1979), extended to accommodate other major international actors including international organizations (e.g., Keohane and Nye 1977; Keohane 1984; Nye 1988). This allows International Relations to make the distinction between domestic or national concerns, which are not the subject of the discipline, and international concerns, which form its core. This distinction is a powerful element in how the discipline has traditionally been constructed. Although few would deny that what happens inside a state can have an impact on relations outside, the domestic/international divide has been a crucial one in determining what is inside the discipline and what is outside.

A key area of investigation is the system in which states operate. Here, orthodox theories are divided over whether the anarchic structure of that system renders the distribution of power the key concern, or whether the system is moderated by rules and norms of behaviour – that is, the degree to which state actions are limited only by relative power (e.g., Mearsheimer 2001), or whether informal rules exist over state behaviour, and whether institutions or regimes can moderate anarchy for mutual benefit (e.g., Bull 1977):

> Revolving in the past around competing theories of human nature, the debate is more concerned today with the extent to which state action is influenced by 'structure' (anarchy and the distribution of power) versus 'process' (interaction and learning) and institutions. Does the absence of centralized political authority force states to play competitive power politics? Can international regimes overcome this logic, and under what conditions? (Wendt 1992: 391)

Because the system remains anarchic, state power is a crucial concern of orthodox accounts. States pursue power not for its own sake, but to promote national interests and, in particular, national security in the context of anarchy.

However, this theoretical divide in International Relations leads to disagreement over whether national interests can best be achieved through cooperation or the competitive maximizing of state power. The latter is emphasized in realist and neo-realist theories. In contrast, neo-liberal theories emphasize the potential for international cooperation to manage insecurity. For both of these theories, however, war and peace have traditionally been the key issues facing the international system; and an ordered system is one without war, rather than one which is just. In this sense, the concerns of the discipline can be seen as a reflection of the interests of its key players. As the discipline grew rapidly after the Second World War, especially in Western Europe and North America, so its concerns reflected the policy interests of states in those regions, notably against the backdrop of the Cold War. In this context, therefore, the first centre of gravity in International Relations concerns what the discipline is about, namely the distinction between domestic and international; a focus on the state as the main actor in the international system; on power, interests and norms as the principles governing how the system works; and on national security and war as the dominant issues of concern for the system and its actors.

The second centre of gravity concerns the nature of theories used in orthodox accounts of International Relations, especially the dominant theories of (neo-)liberalism and (neo-)realism. These theories are based in positivism – that knowledge is advanced through the systematic, and methodologically rigorous, collection of data which then enables the investigator to identify patterns of behaviour. These patterns allow investigators to build theories by inferring the causes behind actions, and to use these theories to predict how subjects might behave (Kurki and Wight 2007: 17, 20–1). For example, in one form of realism, it is inferred that an imbalance of power in the state system is inherently unstable and will lead to war unless a balancing act is undertaken (such as a state increasing its military power or entering into an alliance with another state). The role of theory in this approach is to *explain* the world. Importantly, this world being studied is considered to be 'out there' (external to the observer) and resultant theory is thus seen as separate from the world it is attempting to explain (Hollis and Smith 1991). Orthodox theory also tends towards a form of rationalism, the assumption that behaviour is based upon an assessment by an actor of what is in their best interest. In pursuit of national interests, for instance, it is assumed that governments are aware of, and thus make decisions and act accordingly, based on evaluations of the optimal benefits to the country concerned.

These two centres of gravity in orthodox International Relations – concerning what the discipline is about and the positivist, explanatory and rationalist nature of the theories used – created little space for the consideration of health issues. In particular, health appeared to International Relations scholars as a domestic concern largely unrelated to matters of national security. Although war may impinge on health, both directly through casualties and deaths, and indirectly through its impact on health provision and the creation of new disease risks,[3] these links were considered to be firmly within the realm of health professionals rather than International Relations scholars and policy makers. In other words, because there was no obvious perceived health issue 'out there' for International Relations to explain, there was no requirement for any significant engagement. In this context, a rational assessment was to leave health largely outside of both the discipline of International Relations, and the practice of foreign and security policy.

The principal policy exception to this concerned development aid. Investing in health has been an important part of development policies over the past half-century. This is seen most clearly in the eight high-profile Millennium Development Goals, agreed by the United Nations in 2000, three of which concern health. In addition, eight of its eighteen targets, and eighteen of its forty-eight indicators, also relate directly to health (see section on development in chapter 3). Although development is pursued for humanitarian reasons, it is also closely linked to foreign policy either institutionally or for policy reasons. In the UK, for example, prior to the establishment of the Department for International Development (DfID) in 1997, development aid was under the responsibility of the Foreign and Commonwealth Office (FCO), provided through the Overseas Development Administration. As Baroness Linda Chalker,

Foreign Office Minister responsible for overseas development in the mid-1990s explained, 'Development assistance is part of our broader foreign policy interests' (Chalker 1996). Similarly in the United States, USAID describes its role as 'furthering America's foreign policy interests . . . while improving the lives of citizens in the developing world' (USAID no date).

A second exception has concerned the manner in which health development can be used as part of a 'hearts and minds' approach in strategically important countries. During the Vietnam War, for example, the US military used health interventions called MEDCAPS in an effort to win local support for its operations. In Iraq and Afghanistan, the provision of health assistance has been advocated as part of US counterinsurgency policy (Baker 2007). However, neither the provision of health development assistance nor its use as part of geopolitical strategy has figured prominently on the foreign or security policy agendas of major powers, nor in the core interests of International Relations as an academic discipline except for the occasional crossover with Development Studies.

Interestingly, there are arguably ways in which the subject of health could have been incorporated into the discipline of International Relations, even under the narrow confines of orthodox accounts. For example, a major concern of the discipline is the manner in which rules and norms may mitigate the effects of anarchy within the international system. The discipline is interested in the extent to which states may agree to cooperate out of mutual self-interest, thereby limiting their freedom of action, *despite* the principle of state sovereignty allowing independence of action. Crossborder infectious disease outbreaks provide an excellent example of the tensions between the benefits from, and limitations to, cooperation in a world of sovereign states. It is in the shared interests of all countries that information on the emergence and spread of disease outbreaks is shared openly, but the potential economic and political fallout can lead states to choose to limit the disclosure of information out of national self-interest. This tension emerged during prolonged negotiations from the mid-1990s to revise the International Health Regulations (IHRs), eventually agreed in 2005. The former IHRs, with origins dating from the mid-nineteenth century, oblige states to monitor and report on outbreaks of selected diseases (namely, cholera, plague, yellow fever) within their borders. This obligation was accepted as serving the common good, despite the potential economic and reputational damage such reporting can elicit. Reconciling collective and national interests in the revised IHRs proved a delicate balancing act, with the WHO expanding its ability to call on nongovernmental sources of data but remaining subject to the authority of sovereign states when responding to 'public health emergencies of international concern' (Kamradt-Scott and Lee 2011).

Anarchy might also be mitigated through international institutions and other initiatives. Health has a long and diverse history of international cooperative arrangements, such as the International Sanitary Conferences, International Committee of the Red Cross, and Health Organization of the League of Nations, most designed to promote international norms, establish rules of behaviour and undertake collective action. The WHO was established after the Second World War, as part of the UN system, but remarkably, along with other forms of international health cooperation, remained relatively ignored by International Relations scholars until the early twenty-first century.[4,5] While the organization has remained, for the most part a creature of its member states, there are notable examples of the WHO behaving as an international actor in its own right. This was observed during the SARS epidemic when the WHO not only took the lead in co-ordinating international efforts to combat the outbreak, but issued travel warnings to certain states *despite the wishes of those states*. Overall, health would seem to offer some fertile ground for orthodox scholars of International Relations given the tensions between the requirement for cooperation and the principle of state sovereignty (Kamradt-Scott and Lee forthcoming).

A second way in which health might be expected to feature in International Relations is through human rights. The subject is of interest to the discipline because it poses the question of whether there are certain rights which may be considered universal and, therefore, transcend the sovereignty of states. If this is so, then awkward questions follow over the responsibility of the international community to promote these rights against the wishes and interests of some states and, if these rights are violated, whether the international community has an obligation to act in their defence. Human rights featured prominently during the Cold War when the West[6] was critical of the Eastern bloc's constraints on individual freedoms. During the 1990s, western-led interventions in conflicts such as Bosnia, Kosovo and Sierra Leone were justified by reference to humanitarian values, while criticism of the failure to intervene in the Rwandan conflict was based on genocide being a crime against humanity. What is important for this analysis, however, is that health has been established internationally as a human right, but has largely been ignored in the discussion of human rights by scholars of International Relations despite the right to health being established in a variety of international declarations (see section on human rights in chapter 3).

What these two examples demonstrate is that health *could* have featured more prominently as part of the orthodox agenda for International Relations. The cross/transborder nature of many health issues poses important and interesting questions about the importance of cooperation and the establishment of rules and norms of behaviour. The potential for many diseases to spread between countries, in particular, raises issues about the authority of international organizations, such as the WHO, to act independently of sovereign states. And recognition of health as a universal human right elicits concerns about how they should be promoted and protected within the international community. Moreover, health has featured in both foreign and security policy in the form of development aid for humanitarian and strategic purposes. If the International Relations discipline is in the business of explaining a world 'out there', how could it not have engaged with health issues at these intersections? In other words, the two dominant theories of International Relations fail to account for the relative lack of attention paid to health issues.

This opens up the possibility of a rather different view of the discipline from that outlined above – less a value-neutral explanation of the world and more a discipline which chooses to construct both itself, and the world it seeks to understand, in particular ways. From this perspective, the theories we hold cannot be deemed neutral and divorced from the world they seek to explain or understand; rather they construct or *constitute* that world (e.g., Walker 1993: 6; see also box 2.1). This more reflectivist approach is interested in analysing the meanings and beliefs held by actors. Here, the values, norms and assumptions of those trying to understand the world are important in how we understand the world. The social world is a 'world of our making' (Onuf 1989) and, therefore, reflects our normative prejudices. This does not mean, however, that the material world is of no concern. Adopting a constructivist line, as described in the Introduction, we maintain that the material and ideational worlds closely interact with each other. As Ruggie puts it,

> Constructivists hold the view that the building blocks of international reality are ideational as well as material; that ideational factors have normative as well as instrumental dimensions; that they express not only individual but collective intentionality; and that the meaning and significance of ideational factors are not independent of time and place. (Ruggie 1998: 33)

From the constructivist position, interests are thus not objective givens based on rational analysis of an external reality. Rather they are created inter-subjectively, that is, through an engagement with each other: 'Actors do not have a "portfolio" of interests that they carry around independent of social context; instead, they define their interests in the process of defining situations . . . identities and interests are constituted by collective meanings that are always in process' (Wendt 1992: 398, 407). But, as Smith points out, 'having created [interests] we could create them otherwise; it would be difficult because we have all internalized the "way the world is", but we could make it otherwise' (Smith 2001: 244). Thus an important element of social constructivism is the potential for change in the way in which we understand the world, how we perceive our interests, and ultimately how we behave in it. This change may not be easy because of the way in which our view of the social world is sometimes deeply embedded, but it remains possible. Adopting this position allows us to ask a rather deeper question beyond why health has been largely ignored by International Relations. Instead, our question is based on changing perceptions of interests and understandings. Social constructivism would suggest that health was ignored because interests were not created in a way that allowed them to engage with these questions. The reason for this, we would suggest, had much to do with the bipolar politics of the Cold War, which focused on narrowly defined issues of security, and which created a 'them and us' view of the world, rather than one of commonality in the face of shared threats such as global health risks. As the social context changed with the end of the Cold War, and as the material context changed as well, so perceived interests changed, allowing global health to emerge on the agenda of International Relations. The following section explores this change.

Creating a New Agenda

As described above, International Relations has traditionally been concerned with what the discipline holds as the 'big questions' of war and peace, security and the national interest, a focus matched in foreign policy. In so doing, it removed itself from the daily micro-level questions

---

Box 2.1 Theory and the world

'Theories are part of the social world, they can never be separate from it, and thus they constitute the social world in which we live. Each defines the problems to be examined differently, and we may well define how we know things about those problems in different ways. Thus the social location of the observer will influence which theory they see as most useful, simply because that location will predispose that observer to define some features of international relations as key and others less relevant.' (Smith 2007: 11)

of human survival and well-being, as experienced by millions on the planet struggling with poverty and ill-health. Instead, the discipline focused on the exceptional events affecting the state in its relations with other states. Gradually, however, more critical voices established a foothold linking individual experiences to global forces, and the 'low politics' of basic needs and quality of life to the 'high politics' of the national interest (e.g., Enloe 1989; Thomas, 2000).

Arising from this move were two key ideas which, in turn, developed a degree of purchase in the academic and policy worlds. The first was human security – that security does not simply affect the state, as the referent object, but can be seen from the perspective of the basic needs of individuals. In this sense, the security of the state and the security of individuals are not necessarily one and the same (see section on human security in chapter 6). The second was the idea that both the policy and academic agendas had been too narrowly focused, especially with regard to security, and that a significant broadening was required. New risks such as the environment and climate change, migration and transnational crime began to be articulated as legitimate security concerns for International Relations, alongside the more established concern with military threats and the balance of power. At around the same time, an awareness of the manner in which globalization was affecting world politics began to be emphasized. The speed and intensity of interactions appeared to have increased, and were continuing to increase, creating a change in the pattern of world politics. States appeared to be increasingly subject to broader trends and developments over which they sometimes had only slight control. Within this context, the move to incorporate health into International Relations appears relatively straightforward: health underpins the human security of the individual but is dependent upon increasingly global developments such as the increased mobility of health professionals and patients, international trade agreements affecting access to medicines, and increased population mobility leading to an increased risk of cross/ transborder spread of certain diseases. Equally, the broadening of the agenda created a space which allowed certain health issues, such as bio-terrorism and acute[7] and severe[8] infectious disease outbreaks, to be considered national and global security risks.

Thus, over the past decade, health issues have increasingly featured as part of the academic agenda of International Relations (e.g., Elbe 2009, 2010; Davies 2010) as well as in foreign and security policy (e.g., Downer 2003; Clinton 2010). The change was observable within the policy community from the mid-1990s, but developed more significantly in the early years of the following decade. In 1996 US President

Bill Clinton issued a Presidential Decision Directive calling for a more focused US policy on infectious diseases. This led to a 1999 National Intelligence Estimate on the national security threat from infectious disease (CIA 2000). In 1999 the US Department of State also cited the protection of human health as one of its strategic missions (US State Department 1999: 9, 41). Health issues (and most particularly HIV/AIDS) began to figure prominently in a variety of foreign policy speeches made by key members of the Bush administrations (e.g., Bush 2003; Powell 2004). In its Strategic Plan for Financial Years 2004–9, the US State Department argued that '[t]he United States has a direct interest in safeguarding the health of Americans and in preventing the threats posed by diseases worldwide . . . emerging infectious diseases of epidemic or pandemic proportions . . . pose a serious threat to American citizens and the international community' (US State Department 2004: 76).

In the UK, the Foreign and Commonwealth Office's 2003 strategy paper identified the spread of disease as an ill-effect of globalization, and a risk to peace and development (FCO 2003: 13). Most of the attention in Whitehall to health issues outside of the UK has traditionally come from the DfID, whose 2000 White Paper on International Development also made the link between globalization and poor health (DfID 2000: 21, 34). In Australia, communicable disease was raised (albeit briefly) as a global challenge in its 2003 White Paper on foreign and trade policy (DfAT 2003). Foreign Minister Alexander Downer acknowledged that 'disease and global health issues certainly add to the uncertainty we face in the conduct of our foreign policy' (Downer 2003). One of the clearest statements, in terms of linking health and foreign policy, albeit originating more from within the public health community rather than foreign policy circles, came in the report of the Romanow Commission on *The Future of Health Care in Canada*. The report was critical that 'the broader area of health promotion is very much an afterthought in Canada's foreign policy', and argued that 'we have an opportunity to ensure that access to health care is not only part of our own domestic policy but also a prime objective of our foreign policy as well' (Romanow 2002). Canadian Prime Minister Paul Martin supported the inclusion of health in the Group of 20 (G20) meeting agenda on global challenges, while health issues (again especially HIV/AIDS) appeared prominently on the G8 agenda at Genoa in 2001 and Gleneagles in 2005.

Although there was a small body of scholarly work published in the 1990s, which attempted a link between public health and the sort of concerns that might resonate with International Relations (e.g., Siddiqi

1995; Gordenker 1995), it was at the beginning of the next decade that International Relations scholars began to address health issues as a new part of the discipline's agenda (e.g., Price-Smith 2002; Lee 2003; Elbe 2002, 2003; Prescott 2003). By the end of the decade, articles on health had appeared in most of the leading International Relations journals, a solid number of books had appeared, research councils and other bodies had funded work on the subject of global health and international relations, a number of centres and research programmes had been established across the world,[9] and multiple panels on global health had become a regular feature of the programme of the flagship academic association on the subject, the International Studies Association (ISA), annual convention.

The dominant narrative underpinning this emerging academic and policy agenda can be summarized in three linked moves: that certain health issues led by bio-terrorism and emerging infectious diseases pose new security risks; that the problems are global in scope and not limited to the local or national levels; and that collective action requires a political response going beyond the technical expertise of the public health community and thus engagement with the foreign and security policy community. This narrative, based on perceptions of change in the material world, is important because it constructs a particular view of what is happening and establishes acceptable pathways for response. This not to say that this narrative was the only manner in which International Relations engaged with health issues (e.g., Thomas and Weber 2004), but it did quickly establish a dominant perspective. Nor is it to claim that this was the only major narrative concerning global health apparent at this time. For example, the WHO's Commission on Macroeconomics and Health (CMH), chaired by Harvard economist Jeffrey Sachs who went on to serve as Director of the UN Millennium Project, operated within a different narrative which emphasized the economic value of good health. Crudely put, this narrative suggests that, when individuals are healthy, they are positive contributors to production and consumption which, in turn, encourages economic development and growth. Conversely, when individuals suffer ill-health, the reverse occurs and they became costly drains on an economy. Thus, it was argued that the protection and promotion of population health should be brought under the umbrella of the economic policy of a state. What the CMH further highlighted, however, was that health development was no longer only a national concern but had global implications. Poor health in one area of the world, such as sub-Saharan Africa, could impact elsewhere because of the manner in which the world economy had become globalized (WHO 2001) Moreover, the argument that unhealthy societies that were economically weakened could also become politically unstable brought the argument full circle, thus linking health, economic and foreign policy seamlessly together (Price-Smith 2002). A further narrative marking this new intersection between health and International Relations is focused on biomedical initiatives: diseases can be treated through understanding the nature of viruses and developing better drugs to combat them, but that the globalized nature of the pharmaceutical industry and the speed with which diseases could travel because of increased population mobility means that biomedical research must be approached as a global issue. This narrative, for example, informs the approach of the Bill and Melinda Gates Foundation (BMGF) whose giving power, as described in chapter 5, enables it to influence what normative frames now dominate global health philanthropy.

What is being claimed here is that the manner in which health issues have been incorporated into the International Relations discipline reflects, in large part, a particular dominant narrative or set of narratives emphasizing certain types of risks, the interests of certain population groups, the way in which the global nature of the problem is defined, and the need for certain high-level political responses. But, in so doing, these narratives maintain links with more traditional International Relations concerns. This framing emphasizes, for instance, exceptional events and those which have traction with a national security agenda. Thus, the focus on acute and severe infectious disease outbreaks such as SARS, avian influenza and HIV/AIDS, and on the potential for bio-terrorist attacks, rather than on conditions such as mental health, road traffic accidents, tobacco control and hypertension, which all arguably have global dimensions, reflect these normative frames.[10]

The argument that agendas and interests were not value-neutral givens, or rational responses to external developments, but social constructions allows us to adopt a different perspective. The dominant narrative suggests that International Relations' interest in global health arose from exogenous developments (the emergence of new risks in a globalized environment which required a new form of political response). A more reflectivist position suggests that narratives construct the world in a particular way to emphasize and prioritize certain features over others. These can develop into what we consider a 'normal' or 'commonsensical' way of seeing the world, despite arising from one particular construction of the social world. More critically, it may be argued that narratives serve someone or some purpose. Therefore, rather than a reasoned response to novel developments, this narrative

TABLE 2.1 The top 10 causes of death globally

World	Deaths in millions	Percentage of deaths
Ischaemic heart disease	7.25	12.8
Stroke and other cerebrovascular disease	6.15	10.8
Lower respiratory infections	3.46	6.1
Chronic obstructive pulmonary disease	3.28	5.8
Diarrhoeal diseases	2.46	4.3
HIV/AIDS	1.78	3.1
Trachea, bronchus, lung cancers	1.39	2.4
Tuberculosis	1.34	2.4
Diabetes mellitus	1.26	2.2
Road traffic accidents	1.21	2.1

Source: WHO.

reflects – explicitly or implicitly – a range of interests by privileging certain aspects of global health over others. In this respect, the concern over linking global health to foreign policy, that this might allow one set of policy interests (typically that health policy will become subservient to foreign or security policy goals) to dominate others, is misplaced. Rather, what the dominant narrative does is privilege a series of concerns which are *shared* by *some* health *and* foreign policy communities.

Evidence of the shaping of global health by dominant frames, rather than 'real world' needs, is the disjuncture between the priority given to certain health issues and the actual global burden of death and disease. By most accounts, there is a stark difference between what global health resources are spent on and what actually causes ill-health (see table 2.1).[11] What explains this difference? We explore this question in the following three sections, each of which focuses on one element of this dominant narrative.

Infectious Disease and the New Outbreak Narrative

According to some estimates, infectious diseases account for perhaps one-third (15 million deaths) of total mortality each year, with six diseases (acute respiratory infections, HIV/AIDS, diarrhoeal diseases, malaria, measles and tuberculosis) accounting for 90 per cent of total deaths from infectious disease (e.g., UC Atlas of Global Inequality no date a). As a consequence, it is hardly surprising that infectious diseases receive substantial attention in public health policy. However, two points are worth noting. First, non-communicable diseases cause far higher rates of morbidity and mortality worldwide, killing over 36 million people in 2008 (WHO 2011) yet garner far less scholarly and policy attention. Second, certain infectious diseases, namely acute and severe infections with epidemic potential (e.g., SARS, pandemic influenza, plague) attract far greater notice, including far beyond the public health community, than others which account for a far higher global burden of disease (e.g., acute respiratory infections). What is apparent in contemporary interest in infectious diseases is the need to understand the social construction of such diseases. Central to this is a five-stage narrative (see box 2.2) widely used to explain what has changed and why certain infectious diseases are now considered a major source of global concern.

The significance of this narrative is, not that it tells a story which explains what has happened, but how it shapes our understanding both of what has happened and what is perceived as significant. In other words, it is not a value-neutral account of an exogenous reality, but a particular construction which privileges certain interests and issues over others. Specifically, this new outbreak narrative does four things. First, it tends to privilege acute and severe infectious disease outbreaks (such as SARS and pandemic influenza) over diseases which do not behave in this manner. This may simply be because the mass media find such events newsworthy or, as Leach and Dry (2010) comment, 'chronic is the flipside of exciting' (Leach and Dry 2010: 8). However, this does not seem to provide a full answer. Nor can this be explained by the fact that such diseases cause the highest rates of death and disease. One might alternatively ask, what frames lead to the prioritizing of acute and severe infectious disease outbreaks, and whose interests might be served by this? Equally compelling is the question why non-acute yet severe, or acute but mild, health conditions elicit less notice (see Box 2.2).

Second, it privileges the global over the local. Outbreaks are constructed as global events requiring a co-ordinated response which will be similar across borders. But local differences clearly exist: social ecologies are diverse; health determinants differ from one social context to another; the consequences for different populations vary enormously; and the cultural acceptability of public health measures can change from one society to another. Yet the 'global health' narrative imposes a certain degree of homogeneity with perceived 'universal' values, knowledge and practices being privileged over others. An example is

Box 2.2 The infectious disease narrative

(i) The conquering of infectious disease

Infectious disease is probably as old as humanity itself and for much of our history has been one of the major threats to individual existence. Pandemics such as the Black Death and 1919 Spanish Flu may have been exceptional both in their scale and the numbers affected, but infectious disease appeared to be endemic to the human condition. In the period following the Second World War, however, advances in public health and in drugs, especially antibiotics, appeared to change this, leading the US Surgeon General in the 1960s to declare – probably apocryphally – infectious disease to be conquered. The highpoint of this was the successful eradication of smallpox in 1979 following more than a decade of decline, and for several generations the fear of infectious disease prematurely ending lives receded (at least in developed countries).

(ii) Emerging and re-emerging infectious diseases (ERIDs)

This optimism began to change in the 1990s, although harbingers date back to the previous decade not least with the emergence of the human immuno-deficiency virus (HIV) which first came to prominence in the early 1980s. New diseases began to emerge with unprecedented frequency, by the turn of the millennium averaging one a year. These exploded into public consciousness first with the 2002–3 SARS outbreak, followed by fears over avian flu and then the 2009 outbreak of swine flu. Moreover new, drug resistant forms of diseases believed to be under control began to appear, most notably multi-drug-resistant tuberculosis (MDR-TB) and extensive drug-resistant tuberculosis (EDR-TB). Finally, diseases previously confined to one part of the world began to spread, most notably from Africa to the developed world. These included Ebola and West Nile virus, both of which appeared for the first time in the US in the 1990s. These three developments were all explicitly linked through the use of the term ERIDs, creating the impression of a significant new risk from infectious disease.

(iii) The social ecology of infectious disease

This new and unwelcome development was explained by reference to globally changing patterns of human behaviour. Increased human mobility allowed diseases to be spread quickly into areas previously unaffected. Most dramatic was the advent of so-called 'superspreaders' – individuals infected with a disease who, through their high mobility, could pass the disease on to widely dispersed communities. Increases in urbanization and population density led to increased contact rates, enabling diseases to spread and rapidly maintain a hold on communities. And perhaps finally many of these diseases were zoonotic – that is, originating in the animal kingdom but spreading to humanity – suggesting that the changing relationship with the animal world offered some explanation for the emergence of new diseases. Thus the 2009 H1N1 flu pandemic originated with pigs ('swine flu'); the highly pathogenic influenza A sub-type H5N1 originates in birds, especially chickens ('avian influenza' or 'bird flu') and is associated with humans living in close proximity to chickens usually within an urban environment; and HIV is generally considered to have originated in primates.

Continued

(iv) The increased risk

Key to this narrative is the argument that these new and re-emerging diseases pose an increased risk to individuals, society and economies. The risk to people is in alarmingly high morbidity and mortality rates. This has already been realized with more than 30 million people having died of AIDS-related illnesses, but the potential can also be seen in fears over pandemic influenza. The risk to society is seen most clearly in the case of HIV/AIDS. Fears of high prevalence among the professional and middle classes, especially in some weak and fragile states in sub-Saharan Africa, led organizations ranging from the UN Security Council to think tanks such as the International Crisis Group to worry over the impact on state stability (McInnes 2006, 2007). Concerns were not limited to HIV/AIDS and sub-Saharan Africa, however. The potential for pandemic influenza to disrupt the functioning of industrial and post-industrial states has been highlighted by the World Bank (e.g., Burns et al. 2008). Finally these diseases pose risks to economies through disrupting trade and preventing people from going to work (either because they are ill, fear becoming ill, are prevented by quarantine measures from attending work, or cannot get to work because of disruption to transport infrastructure). The economic cost of the SARS outbreak has been estimated as several tens of billions of dollars, despite the fact that fewer than 10,000 cases were reported and fewer than 1,000 people died of the disease. This indicates the potential for not only disease but fear of disease to disrupt economies. Indeed, it is widely believed that the British and American governments placed pressure on the World Health Organization not to declare swine flu a pandemic because of fears over the economic impact at a time when the global economy was facing recession through the banking crisis.

(v) Response

Priscilla Wald identifies a particular 'outbreak narrative' as constructing public health's understanding of how to respond to disease. This involves an established methodology consisting of: disease surveillance leading to outbreak alerts; the development of vaccines and an understanding of the disease's epidemiology; and finally the control of disease through drugs and public health measures (Wald 2007). The new narrative which we identify goes further than this, however, advocating the need for increased international cooperation and improved global health governance measures, especially over surveillance and disease control. In other words, what has happened is that in this narrative the emergence of new diseases coupled to increased risks has led to the requirement for more than a technocratic response involving better public health measures. Rather what was needed was better health governance at a global level.

the 'ABC' campaign[12] (which stands for abstinence, being tested and being faithful in marriage and monogamous relationships, and the correct and consistent use of condoms for those who practice high-risk behaviours) to prevent the spread of HIV/AIDS in Africa. The strategy was adopted by international organizations such as UNAIDS, as well as major initiatives such as the US President's Emergency Plan for AIDS Relief (PEPFAR). The campaign, however, has been widely criticized for applying Western-based values and, more precisely, conservative Christian beliefs about morality (in particular, PEPFAR's reluctance to promote condom use was seen as testament to the primacy given to religious beliefs rather than public health evidence), in social settings where, for instance, women were often unable to negotiate safe sex, where transactional sex may be a necessary survival strategy, or where condom use may have cultural taboos (Dietrich 2007). Indeed, the tendency to portray the disease as the same across societies led UNAIDS to react by arguing 'know your epidemic' in developing effective HIV prevention programming – that HIV/AIDS is not a pandemic but a series of epidemics with different causes and consequences across different societies.[13] Similarly, during the H1N1 influenza pandemic in 2009, concern over the potential role of pigs in spreading the virus led to mass culling in some countries. When this was carried out in Egypt however, the impact on the minority Christian population was disproportionate. Additionally, pigs are an important mechanism for waste disposal in the country, and culling had knock-on effects for public health from the accumulation of rubbish (Tadros 2010).

Third, the outbreak narrative focuses on the 'downstream' treatment of disease and control of its further spread, rather than prevention of diseases occurring in the first place by tackling 'upstream' socioeconomic and environmental causes. This is manifest in a concern with treatments in response to outbreaks through the strengthening of diagnostics, 'surge capacity' to deal with increased case loads, and the development of drugs to treat patients. Disease prevention, with the exception of vaccine development and application, in contrast, is given relatively short shrift. Thus, the H1N1 influenza pandemic, and fears of a more severe H5N1 pandemic, saw a focus on rapid case detection, creating stockpiles to ensure the availability of the anti-viral drugs, social distancing and quarantining of infected individuals, and the development and use of vaccines to prevent further spread. The contribution of intensive farming methods, patterns of human and animal co-habitation, and other socioeconomic factors that increase the risk of influenza pandemics arising remain little addressed. Perhaps the most noteworthy exception to this was the emphasis on abstinence as a means of controlling the spread of HIV in Africa, an approach advocated by the Bush administration in the US. However, the motivation for this appeared to be based less on empirical evidence supporting the effectiveness of such a policy (which was somewhat lacking), and more on the privileging of certain mores based on conservative religious beliefs which were influential in the US at that time (see Busby 2007; Ingram 2007, 2010).

Finally, the narrative develops an 'inside/outside' dichotomy, where infectious disease outbreaks are seen as threats emanating from 'outside' western countries or 'over there' in the developing world. Thus, the narrative emphasizes the origin of emerging diseases as Asia (SARS and avian influenza), Africa (Ebola, HIV/AIDS, West Nile virus) or Latin America (cholera, pandemic influenza). The primary populations cast as 'at risk', within this narrative, are western societies. There is thus more than a whiff of colonial assumptions over backward customs and insanitary lifestyles (see Leach and Dry 2010) seen also in the Bush administration's emphasis on abstinence as a means of controlling HIV. What this element of the narrative does, in short, is place blame on the external, legitimizing a privileging of western interests as threatened, and downplaying any contribution that western societies may play in creating and maintaining the structural conditions by which such outbreaks occur.[14]

Growing attention to non-communicable diseases (NCDs), as indicated by the UN High Level Meeting on Non-communicable Diseases in 2011, suggests a potential challenge to the dominance of the outbreak narrative. How the problem of NCDs has been framed to date, however, may indicate an extension of, rather than an overturning of this dominant narrative. The use of language reminiscent of infectious disease outbreaks, such as 'pandemic' and 'vectors', to describe NCDs (Brock et al. 2007) has been used to create greater urgency in tackling these conditions. The stronger emphasis on downstream clinical treatments, such as beta blockers (to treat hypertension), statins (to lower cholesterol), insulin (to regulate blood sugar in diabetes), rather than upstream changes in the form of health promotion, is also telling (Cohen 2011). What conditions, in the gamut of NCDs now facing modern societies, will and will not be given priority, and how they are eventually addressed, will reveal the extent to which a genuine shift in framing global health issues has occurred.

In conclusion, this contemporary outbreak narrative constructs a particular view of the world by offering an explanation of what is happening and, by so doing, privileges certain ideas, interests and institutions. It privileges the powerful through an emphasis on certain diseases which most threaten their interests. There are diseases which cause higher rates of morbidity and mortality but, as they are largely confined to populations without such power, they receive more limited attention. In turn, the resultant agenda privileges certain types of methodologies and policy responses.

'Health is Global'

That health has an international dimension is well established, although definitions and understandings of 'international health' also vary – from crossborder health issues, to health in the ex-colonized or broader developing world, to health problems simply 'elsewhere' from a given domestic context. During the nineteenth century, fears that cholera and other epidemic diseases would impact adversely on burgeoning political and economic links between imperialist powers and their expanding domains led to the convening of the International Sanitary Conferences. This marked the birth of international health, as it became known, and the term remained in general use for almost all of twentieth century. By the 1990s, however, a shift in terminology from 'international' to 'global' health, as discussed in chapter 1, began to be visibly apparent. The Institute of Medicine (1997) set out 'America's vital interest in global health' (see also Fidler and Drager 2009) and, by 2008, the UK Department of Health had produced a policy statement entitled *Health is Global*, arguing that a national perspective on health policy was no longer adequate, given that health was now subject to global forces (Department of Health 2008a). What has emerged is a dominant consensus that health is no longer a predominately national-level concern (with some limited international relevance), but has significant global dimensions. This qualitative shift in the nature of health determinants and outcomes, including the production of health care (goods and services), has led to diverse calls for better global health governance, given the limits placed on national governance frameworks by globalization (see, e.g., Cooper et al. 2009). David Fidler has gone further, arguing that this shift from national to global health governance is already in motion, as illustrated by the WHO's role in the SARS outbreak. He argues that the organization's overriding of the wishes of sovereign member states, in issuing travel warnings, demonstrated its emergence as a body capable of supranational powers, and that this heralded a post-Westphalian era in health governance (Fidler 2003, 2004). However, the empirical evidence, not only for Fidler's claim but for the wider global health argument, is more equivocal. Leach and Dry (2010), for example, identify the enduring importance of local practices and variations in health care, while Frank Smith (2010) persuasively argues that the response to the 2009 influenza pandemic was informed by national interests rather than global health governance. In other words, many health issues remain local and the pursuit of national interests suggests the continued potency of sovereign states, rather than a decisive movement, towards a post-Westphalian system (see box 2.3).

A strict assessment of the alleged shift, from international to global health, and from international to global health governance thus seems warranted. This might be achieved, for example, through the work of the International Relations theorist Jan Aarte Scholte, as described in chapter 1, who offers a relatively strict definition of 'globalization' as deterritorialization. That the social construction of the term global health has been based on a far looser and broader concept of global, to date, is in itself important to interrogate. Globalization and global

Box 2.3 The limits of globalization

It has become commonplace to argue that infectious disease knows no borders and that, although the potential for infectious disease to spread across communities is hardly new, increased globalization has created a new environment where disease can spread more quickly and more easily than before. This move has been critical in establishing health as global. From a reflectivist position, however, what is important is the fact that analysts have chosen to emphasize the extent of globalization leading to increased risk from infectious disease. But there are limits to the extent to which infectious disease can be considered 'global'. Even if a disease spreads to become a pandemic, the capacity to protect and promote population health is far from global. Responses to disease may and usually do vary from state to state because of a variety of factors. A key difference may be wealth – rich states may be able to afford vaccines and advanced health care, while poorer states may not. This was seen in the 2009 influenza pandemic where some states such as the UK were able to purchase large quantities of the drug Tamiflu, despite the numbers of cases being relatively small, while poorer states were not able to do so despite a potentially greater risk. Responses may also vary because of cultural or religious factors. Condoms are a proven defence against the spread of HIV/AIDS, and have been widely promoted for this purpose in a large number of states, including the UK and US. The Catholic Church, however, has historical concerns over condom use because of its birth control properties, while some African societies see condom use as 'unmanly'.

Less attention grabbing but no less political is the manner in which government control can be exercised over populations during epidemics. If a disease spreads by human-to-human contact, then minimizing such contact will slow or even prevent the spread of disease. This policy of social distancing runs against liberal values of free association, some of which may be enshrined in constitutions. Even when they do not receive this level of formal support, norms of free association may be strong in some states. Social distancing measures may therefore be difficult to introduce in these states, and resistance may be strong. In more authoritarian states, however, it may be easier to impose such measures because of the political system of these states. The point here then is not to deny that disease may spread internationally, but that the health effects are national and that health responses are nationally conditioned.

health have come to form an important element in the dominant narrative identified above and, in so doing, serve certain interests, practices and forms of knowledge over others. What interests are served by specific definitions of global health? How do such interests benefit from the particular way the globalization of health issues has been articulated?

The Politicization of Global Health

The final element of this dominant narrative is perhaps the most obviously controversial. Traditionally, political interference in the health field has been resisted, at least as an ideal. It is often prescriptively argued that the making of health policy, ranging from the individual clinician to global health initiatives, should be based on factually-based (value-neutral) clinical evidence of health need, rather than any politically pre-determined (value-based) priority. Most health care professionals are bound by some form of the Hippocratic Oath which commits them to a duty of care to all patients. The Declaration of Geneva, originally adopted by the World Medical Association in 1948 and subsequently amended most recently in 2006, for example, states that health professionals will 'not permit considerations of age, disease or disability, creed, ethnic origin, gender, nationality, political affiliation, race, sexual orientation, social standing or any other factor to intervene' in his/her duty to a patient (see box 2.4). Similarly, the Geneva Conventions require parties in war, and occupying powers, to provide medical care to wounded prisoners and civilians. In this sense, it is widely held that health should be accorded the highest normative value, taking precedence over other value systems.

In practice, however, this certainly does not mean that politics does not play a part in the health field. The allocation of limited resources by governments to the health sector, and within the health sector to a broad range of health needs, as well as decisions on how such resources will be used to deliver health care and to whom, are ultimately questions with strong political dimensions. The answers to these questions are not wholly resolvable by factual evidence, but invariably encompass normative assumptions. Even decisions about how 'need' is defined in health policy, whether by conditions requiring most urgent treatment, by the likelihood of successful treatment, by the availability of cost-effective interventions, or even by populations deemed most economically beneficial to wider society, entail value-based judgements. If politics is fundamentally about who gets what, then the normative basis underpinning health policy decisions are political.

Box 2.4 The Declaration of Geneva

The Declaration was originally adopted by the General Assembly of the World Medical Assembly at its 1948 meeting in Geneva and was subsequently revised in 1968, 1984, 1994, 2005 and 2006.

- I solemnly pledge to consecrate my life to the service of humanity;
- I will give to my teachers the respect and gratitude that is their due;
- I will practice my profession with conscience and dignity;
- The health of my patient will be my first consideration;
- I will respect the secrets that are confided in me, even after the patient has died;
- I will maintain by all the means in my power, the honor and the noble traditions of the medical profession;
- My colleagues will be my sisters and brothers;
- I will not permit considerations of age, disease or disability, creed, ethnic origin, gender, nationality, political affiliation, race, sexual orientation, social standing or any other factor to intervene between my duty and my patient;
- I will maintain the utmost respect for human life;
- I will not use my medical knowledge to violate human rights and civil liberties, even under threat;
- I make these promises solemnly, freely and upon my honor.

Source: World Medical Association (2006)

The perspective that health politics is a necessary evil, that should be minimized at all costs, is reflected in two main framings (see box 1.4) of health policy following the Second World War: the evidence-based medicine and rights-based frames. The former broadly views health as a technical problem where the gathering of certain types of factual evidence (with the randomized control trial as the gold standard of such evidence) can lead to the identification of universal lessons and 'best practice'. This approach covers the working of the human body to patterns of health and disease within populations. A good example is cardiovascular disease (CVD) for which the accumulation of evidence across many patients and numerous studies has identified a series of individual risk factors. The World Heart Federation, for example, identifies tobacco use, alcohol use, high blood pressure (hypertension), high cholesterol, obesity, physical inactivity and unhealthy diets as the main risk factors for coronary heart disease and stroke.[15] How the problem of CVD is defined, and thus what the possible solutions are, focus on the need for individual behavioural change and the medical treatment of related conditions (such as statins to lower cholesterol and beta blockers to treat hypertension). This approach, however, gives far less attention to the structural factors which lead to such behaviours, including socioeconomic status, changing work conditions, discrimination and social stigma, urban design and corporate marketing practices. To a large extent, in other words, the evidence-based medicine frame tends to depoliticize health, emphasizing individual behaviour and, by extension responsibility for personal decisions and actions, and de-emphasizing the social context within which people make health-related choices.

In this context, politics is not only seen as unnecessary, but considered a hindrance or interference in rational decision making. At best, politics muddies the water by preventing objective assessment, based on scientific (value-neutral) evidence, and at worst it can lead to disastrous policies. An often cited example of the latter was the manner in which Thabo Mbeki, when serving as President of South Africa, dismissed the connection between HIV and AIDS, arguing that this was a ploy to force his country into buying expensive anti-retrovirals to treat those infected with the virus. His health minister, Manto Tshabalala-Msimang, promoted cheaper alternatives, such as beetroot and garlic, based on ideas rooted in traditional medicine. A large part of this policy can be understood politically: as a post-colonial discourse of an African nation wishing to resist continued Western domination, on this occasion through Western bio-medical practices. The result was condemned by the scientific medical community, and almost certainly led to unnecessary suffering and loss of life from HIV/AIDS in South Africa. This is seen as an example of how politics can interfere with rational evidence-based health policy.

The rights-based approach takes a similar view that political interference is damaging to health policy. According to this approach, health is seen as beyond politics and based instead upon natural law (that is, a universalist sense of moral behaviour). In so doing, of course, it may be argued that this is in itself a political construction in privileging certain rights, and indeed to promote rights per se. For the most part, however, the rights-based approach is seen rather differently, as being in some sense superior to, and thus trumping, more narrowly based politics. The approach can be found in a wide range of international legal documents over the past sixty years, including the preamble to the 1948 Constitution of the WHO, with 'the enjoyment of the highest attainable standard of health' as 'one of the fundamental rights of every human being' (WHO 1946 amended 2006); the 1978 Declaration of Alma Ata on the right to primary health care (see box 3.6); and the Millennium Development Goals (MDGs) (see box 3.4). In all of these, health is portrayed as a superordinate goal, and political interference can only undermine the rights of individuals to attain a basic level of health.[16] It is an approach associated with international development, of poverty relief, and improving the human condition, rather than one linked to power politics and the pursuit of interests.

Since 2000, however, two further frames have proved increasingly influential, both of which place politics more obviously within the arena of global health. The first was economism, which emphasized health as part of a collective good. The origins of this approach lay as a reaction to the neo-liberal paradigm which dominated public policy during the 1980s onwards in many countries. The starkest advocates of neo-liberalism in health policy stressed the efficiency of the market in distributing health resources and delivering health care, viewing patients as consumers exercising rational choice to maximize benefits. Neo-liberalism's influence was seen not only in the reform policies of the US, UK and other major western countries, but in the policies of key international institutions such as the International Monetary Fund (IMF) and World Bank. Moreover, this approach claimed to be resistant to political interference, arguing that unleashing the rationalism of competitive market forces would produce the greatest good for the greatest numbers in society. Allowing politics to 'interfere' with the market, however, would lead to less than optimal levels of benefit.

By the end of the 1990s, however, this approach was being challenged by a more Keynesian approach to health policy. As described above, the report of the WHO Commission on Macroeconomics and Health proved to be highly influential. Sachs argued that the disease burden on the poor threatened the health, and thus wealth, of individual societies (WHO 2001). Investment in the health needs of developing countries was needed as a core component of their economic growth and development strategies. Furthermore, and in the context of rapidly growing concern with 'global health', such investments were needed to prevent spillover effects threatening regional or even global well-being. This approach directly informed the setting and pursuit of the MDGs:

> The Millennium Development Goals depend critically on scaling up public health investments in developing countries. As a matter of urgency, developing-country governments must present detailed investment plans that are sufficiently ambitious to meet the goals, and the plans must be inserted into existing donor processes. Donor countries must keep the promises they have often reiterated of increased assistance, which they can easily afford, to help improve health in the developing countries and ensure stability for the whole world. (Sachs 2004: 947)

Thus, in contrast to neo-liberalism, which argues for minimal state interference in markets, Sachs argued in favour of such interference.

A second more political frame was securitization through the linkage between health, and foreign and security policy. As described above, these two realms have historically been seen as occupying distinct realms, with health policy operating at the national level and inwardly domestic looking, and foreign and security policy focused outward at the international level. Since the 1990s, links have been increasingly drawn between the two by the scholarly and policy communities. Moreover, these links have become bi-directional in that both communities have seen benefit in making them. This has led to the coining and promotion of such concepts as 'global health security' and 'global heath diplomacy' (see chapters 3 and 6), and to a variety of initiatives to further their mutuality. To some extent, this interest can be seen as part of the broadening of the post-Cold War 'new security' agenda, as described previously, and a response to a perceived 'clear and present danger' arising especially from acute and severe infectious disease outbreaks and bio-terrorism in the wake of the attacks on the World Trade Center on 11 September 2001 (McInnes and Lee 2006; Elbe 2010). Neither of these fears, however, has been supported empirically: the number of bio-terrorist attacks has actually reduced since 9/11 while infectious disease outbreaks have yet to lead to any national security crises or state collapse.

An alternative argument might be that the link was socially constructed by a number of opinion formers in the health and foreign policy communities as a means of garnering greater attention to a series of emergent public health crises. How successful such efforts have been remain unclear. It is not clear, for example, that increases in health development aid have been directly driven by security or foreign policy concerns (see, e.g., McInnes and Rushton 2010). What is important, and the focus of this book, is the need to understand the coming together of global health and International Relations as something more than a contestation over material interests. We argue that the terrain of contestation is over the 'big ideas' that frame the two realms, and that it is the construction and reconstruction of specific narratives, such as described above, that has shaped the politics of global health over the past two decades.

Conclusion

At the turn of the millennium, a new agenda began to appear linking global health and International Relations. This agenda has reflected a desire to cut across existing boundaries, in both the academic and policy worlds, to address perceived pressing needs. Central to this agenda has been the development of a narrative focusing on the emergence of acute and severe infectious disease outbreaks, the global nature of health, and an increased emphasis on health as a political arena. For many, the development and promotion of this agenda has been welcome – the world had changed; new risks (and to a lesser extent possibilities) had emerged most often linked to globalization; and a new relationship was needed between the two hitherto separate fields to explain what was happening and to address these changes.

The emergence of this new agenda has by no means been unproblematic, with concerns being expressed not least over health being subjugated to the more *realpolitik* perspectives of foreign and security policy (see, e.g., Elbe 2006). What is striking is how little critical engagement there has been over the relationship between global health and International Relations, and the agenda which it has promoted. The relationship has generally been presented either as rational and desirable, while the few critics of the link have generally worried over the potential negative impact it might have on recent political gains for health.[17] Throughout there has been an underlying sense that the link has been a natural 'coming together' prompted by exogenous pressures, and that the key issue is how to make this new relationship work best.

This chapter takes a more reflexive line. Its central argument is that this emergent agenda is not 'natural' or 'rational', but constructed around particular narratives which privilege certain interests, ideas and institutions over others. Why, for example, have certain types of infectious disease outbreaks been prioritized when the vast majority of deaths worldwide come from non-communicable diseases? Why are biomedical determinants of health recognized as 'global', and given greater weight in health policy and research, while the global dimensions of the social determinants of health continue to struggle to gain political traction? Indeed, why does global health continue to defy definition amid unprecedented attention to the subject?

From this perspective, there is less that is new and radical about this agenda than might initially appear to be the case. While we agree with other commentators that the recent development of a mutual interest between global health and International Relations is both novel and noteworthy, the interests this agenda promotes may not be. As played out to date, the global health agenda does not envisage a radical reordering of the social world to prioritize those most in need, but remains largely focused on dominant interests that hold material and ideational power. The remainder of this book explores this core argument as an important step towards a critical understanding of the contemporary nature of global health and International Relations theory and practice.

CHAPTER THREE

Health, Foreign Policy and Global Health Diplomacy

In a seminal 2004 article, David Fidler commented that public health in the twenty-first century had undergone a revolution. This revolution was not technical in nature – that is, in the form of improved treatments or practices – but political. In Fidler's (2004: 45) words, 'the previously obscure and neglected policy area of public health shed obscurity and neglect to become the subject matter of intense national and homeland security, foreign policy, and global governance debates'. In writing this, Fidler was reflecting a growing sentiment that something dramatic had happened in the relationship between health and foreign policy. In 1999 WHO Director-General, Gro Harlem Brundtland, had addressed the prestigious Council on Foreign Relations in New York on 'Why investing in global health is good politics', arguing that the world had changed and that furthering national interests in health requires international (i.e. inter-state) cooperation: 'with globalization – on which this nation's prosperity so much depends – all of humankind today paddles in a single microbial sea – and we have to conclude: there are no health sanctuaries' (Brundtland 1999: 2). Brundtland's initiative had sparked a decade of rumbling controversy over whether the WHO should take a more overt 'political' role, working with foreign policy elites, to strengthen international cooperation on global health issues (e.g., Møgedal and Alveberg 2010), or whether it should focus on its 'core competencies', most often defined in terms of technical advice and standards setting (e.g., Reeves and Brundage 2011). Her speech had also laid the ground over the next five years for a number of statements and initiatives, from foreign policy leaders, drawing a link between health and foreign policy. By the second half of the decade the inclusion of health issues in foreign policy statements was, if not commonplace, then at least unexceptional (see, e.g., McInnes and Lee 2006).

This period was also marked by the emergence of the term 'global health diplomacy'. By the end of the decade, global health diplomacy was in extensive use, especially within the public health community, reflecting a growing desire to facilitate international cooperation to address pressing global health issues. The rationale for turning to diplomacy was that many health issues, and their determinants, were seen as no longer bound by the territorial borders of the state, as described in the previous chapter. Governments, along with the multitude of institutional actors now active in the global health arena, needed to work more closely together. Negotiating what this collective action would be, and the institutional arrangements by which it would be carried out (see the discussion of global health governance in chapter 5), fell within the province of diplomacy.

Despite widespread support for global health diplomacy, how the term has been used has remained somewhat vague, encompassing almost any relationship between foreign policy and global health, and even contradictory within the scholarly literature and policy circles (Feldbaum and Michaud 2010: 1). Fidler (2011: 5) notes that definitions are 'all over the map', while Lee and Smith (in press) argue that 'the term has largely been used normatively to describe its expected purpose rather than distinct features.' Novotny and Kickbusch (2009: 41) reveal a further conceptual challenge when they refer to the potentially contradictory 'dual goals' of global health diplomacy, in advancing either public health or strengthening foreign policy. Much of the existing global health diplomacy literature maintains a strong normative dimension, namely the furthering of a healthier world, rather than a more *realpolitik* line of advancing states' interests. However, this is a reflection of the origins of this literature within public health circles, rather than any clear reconciliation of the two policy communities.

Within this context, one key initiative linking health and foreign policy was announced in 2006 when the ministers of foreign affairs from France, Indonesia, Norway, Senegal, South Africa and Thailand announced the commencement of a process of cooperation on health and foreign policy. The disparate nature of this grouping is one of the key reasons for its significance, demonstrating how the link can cut across geographical, religious and economic barriers. The centrepiece of this cooperative arrangement is the 'Oslo Declaration', which argues that 'health is one of the most important . . . foreign policy issues of our time' (Oslo Declaration 2007: 1373; see also Møgedal and Alveberg 2010). The Oslo Declaration was acknowledged by the UN General Assembly, where Resolution 64/108 'recognized the close relationship between global health and foreign policy' (UNGA 2010: 3). Despite being a non-member of the Oslo group, the link was also affirmed by the US government. In 2009 President Barack Obama launched his Global Health Initiative, echoing Brundtland's words from a decade previously, arguing that '[w]e cannot wall ourselves off from the world and hope for the best, nor ignore the public health challenges beyond our borders' (White House 2009). US Secretary of State Hillary Clinton (2010) similarly declared that the 'long standing commitment to global health' was a 'signature of American leadership in the world today'.

This change, however, was constructed by Fidler and others (e.g., Feldbaum et al. 2010; Oslo Declaration 2007: 1373), not as two previously distinct policy areas suddenly encountering each other for the first time, but as a change in both the nature and intensity of a relationship which stretched back at least into the nineteenth century. Originally, these links were born out of the expansion of trade, especially between Europe and the rest of the world. With increased trade came the risk of diseases spreading to Europe. Trade was itself a vector for disease and therefore represented an exogenous threat to European countries. Yet it was also an essential driver of European economic growth and prosperity, and was potentially threatened by measures to protect public health. This tension between the promotion of trade and protection of health could not be resolved at the national level. Instead international cooperation was sought, resulting in the negotiation of a series of conventions on trade and health, the International Sanitary Conventions. Thus public health encountered foreign policy through the need to mitigate the risks to health from increased trade. Foreign policy encountered public health through the need to mitigate the risks to trade from increased epidemics.

At the end of the Second World War, however, this narrowly circumscribed relationship expanded somewhat, from a focused concern with trade relations, to human rights and development. Central to this narrative is that development and human rights were deemed peripheral to both health and foreign policy after the Second World War. Although both featured at times within foreign policy, they were generally considered as part of the meta-narrative of Cold War competition rather than ends in themselves. While health in the industrialized world steadily improved in the decades following the Second World War, thanks to better living conditions and health care, good health within the poorest countries continued to be a constant struggle for most. The link between poverty and ill-health was firmly established and international health cooperation became constructed as a development problem albeit addressed often along Cold War lines (Fidler 2004: 45–72). The founders of the WHO adopted the idea of health as a human right in the preamble to the WHO Constitution, an idea reiterated during the 1970s with the Health for All movement and Declaration of Alma Ata (see section below on human rights and box 3.5). However, the organization subsequently retreated towards a technocratic approach to health cooperation which focused on disease control and standards setting, rather than thornier issues such as social justice and the reallocation of resources.

By the early 1990s, it was not the end of the Cold War that appears to have prompted change in the relationship between health and foreign policy, although events may have provided a permissive atmosphere for a different relationship. Rather, globalization and the interconnectedness of health issues in a global village was identified as the key agent of change (e.g., Brundtland 1999; McMichael and Beaglehole 2000; Fidler 2004; Lee 2004). Much of the attention in this narrative focused on familiar fears but writ large, namely trade relations increasing the spread of emerging and re-emerging diseases. These risks were recognized as greater in the late twentieth century given the intensity of population movements, trade of goods and services, flows of information and communication, and unprecedented impacts on local and global environments. Like the imperialist powers of the nineteenth century, countries at the forefront of globalization perceived themselves especially vulnerable to new health risks, including the resurgence of infectious disease outbreaks, fears that had largely retreated from high-income countries (Garrett 1994). Other, albeit fewer, writers identified opportunities from globalization in the increased availability of treatments, the spread of knowledge and the more widespread promotion of rights (Institute of Medicine 1997: 7; McMichael and Beaglehole 2000; Colgan 2002: 8; Oslo Declaration 2007: 1374).

Dissenters to this narrative were few. Stuart Harris, for example, noted that, although much of foreign policy has health implications, the relationship was a 'marriage of convenience' with little inter-marital conversation (Harris 2004: 171–2). What is also noteworthy is that the dominant narrative was one which narrowly emphasized the threat of infectious disease outbreaks to high-income countries, as described in chapter 2, rather than the threat to low- and middle-income countries, the impact on other health conditions beyond infectious disease outbreaks, or the nature of economic globalization and trade liberalization as the core problem. For example, the new risks from non-communicable diseases associated with the increased global production and consumption of food high in fat, salt and sugar, tobacco and alcohol, and changing patterns of work; the worldwide impacts of privatization and deregulation on health services and financing; and the effects of globalization on patterns of mental health, road traffic accidents, violence and injuries, work-related injuries and deaths, and the health effects of exposure to dangerous substances were given limited attention. This is not to say that these latter risks were wholly ignored.

Indeed, arguably one of the greatest triumphs of this new relationship was the signing of the Framework Convention on Tobacco Control (FCTC) in 2003, while agreement on the Millennium Development Goals (MDGs) in 2000 reinvigorated development policies. But the agenda was dominated by the threat of infectious disease outbreaks spreading to high-income countries. Fidler (2004: 87) reflects this agenda in commenting:

> Infectious diseases are framed as exogenous threats to the foreign policy interests and national security of the great powers. The heightened risk of disease importation by developed countries in the era of globalization represents a direct exogenous threat that the literature on emerging infectious diseases repeatedly emphasized. The negative consequences of disease-exacerbated political and economic problems in developing countries constitute an indirect exogenous threat infectious diseases pose for developed states. The policy advice urges the great powers to reduce their vulnerability to the direct and indirect exogenous threats by exercising their material power in ways that mitigate these threats.

In a similar vein, the US Institute of Medicine (1997: 3–4) argued that 'America has a vital and direct stake in the health of people around the globe', but that 'America must engage in the fight for global health from its strongest basis: its pre-eminence in science and technology'. This was interpreted as a focus on controlling external disease threats to protect US interests, especially infectious diseases, through the development (and even export) of drug treatments and clinical interventions. On the use of US political and economic power to address the harmful health effects to all populations from tobacco, certain food and drink products, toxic substances, environmental degradation, working conditions or health worker migration, the report was virtually silent.

This chapter identifies six main points of intersection in the debate linking health and foreign policy – that is, those issues which are constructed as part of the agenda – and describes how the narratives underpinning these intersections have privileged certain ideas, interests and institutions over others. It also attempts to identify how that agenda is prioritized and whom it benefits. One way in which the debate has been constructed is over whether this cooperation should primarily benefit health or foreign policy. In an idealized situation both would benefit. But the question is not simply which is prioritized when the two are in conflict, but how the relationship has been constructed to privilege one over the other (see boxes 3.1 and 3.2). The debate is, thus, not simply about which sphere should be prioritized, health or foreign policy, but about broader interests in a globalized world which may transcend national boundaries and hence the confines of traditional foreign

Box 3.1 Making foreign policy work for health: Global health diplomacy as health promotion

Despite its vague and often contradictory meanings, one common use of the term global health diplomacy has been to describe how health needs to utilize diplomacy in an era of globalization. Lee and Gomez (2011: 62) reflect this approach, arguing that global health diplomacy is 'a way of harnessing foreign policy actors and processes for the benefit of global health good'. Drager and Fidler (2007: 162) similarly argue that '[c]ritical to global health diplomacy is the relationship between health and foreign policy. Even though much of what affects health today is transnational in nature, countries remain core actors that must reorient their health and foreign policies in ways that align their national interests with the diplomatic, epidemiological and ethical realities of a globalized world'. From a foreign policy background, Keri-Ann Jones (2010: 1) of the US State Department argues that 'International diplomatic engagement is essential to building global policies to address health issues'. The key examples usually cited as successes of global health diplomacy are the Framework Convention on Tobacco Control (FCTC) and the revision of the International Health Regulations (IHRs). Both involved states and other international actors working together to produce an agreement to advance public health. But other examples also exist. Chan, Chen and Xu (2010) demonstrate how China has started to use global health diplomacy after the SARS outbreak, Ozdemir et al. (2009) use it to argue for greater governance in the use of genomics for personalized medicine, and Lee and Gomez (2011: 62) cite the 2005 Paris Declaration on Aid Effectiveness as an example.

Box 3.2 Using health to advance foreign policy: Health as soft and smart power

In 1990 Joseph S. Nye identified a shift away from traditional measures of power in foreign policy – military strength, population, geography and resources – and the methods of exploiting these based on coercion and payment. Instead, he argued that 'soft power' was becoming increasingly important, where the measures of power were culture, values and institutions and the methods coption and attraction (Nye 1990). Since then Nye has clarified his position, suggesting that both traditional hard power and soft power need to be used in conjunction as smart power: 'soft power is the ability to obtain preferred outcomes through attraction. If a state can set the agenda for others or shape their preferences, it can save a lot on carrots and sticks. But rarely can it replace either. Thus the need for smart strategies that combine the tools of both hard and soft power' (Nye 2009: 160).

The potential for health as a tool of soft power has been recognized by a number of states. Although China has a longstanding development aid commitment to Africa, Youde also identifies the manner in which China has used health to gain influence there. It has sent medical personnel, donated drugs and provided equipment to African states both as development assistance but also as part of a policy to improve its standing on the continent. But as Youde points out, this is not a targeted strategy with a clearly defined outcome in mind: 'No African ambassador would proclaim in the United Nations General Assembly that it was voting with the People's Republic of China because the Chinese government had announced the shipment of one million anti-malarial doses' (Youde 2010a: 160). Instead this is a long-term strategy aimed to create a favourable view of China: 'Indeed, it is entirely plausible that members of a government may not necessarily connect their favourable views of China to elements of soft power' (Youde 2010a: 160). In a similar vein, Feinsilver (2009) notes how Cuba has been conducting 'medical diplomacy' since 1960, provid-ing both medical assistance to scores of developing countries, some on a long-term basis, and free medical education to tens of thousands of foreign students. In so doing it 'has garnered symbolic capital (prestige, good will and influ-ence) . . . beyond what would otherwise have been possible and has helped cement Cuba's role as a player on the world stage' (Feinsilver 2009: 273). In the US, former majority leader Senator William H. Frist, himself a medical doctor, suggested that medicine could act 'as a currency of peace' (Frist 2008). The influential Washington-based think tank produced a report on *Smart Global Health Policy* which argues that 'Americans have long understood that promot-ing global health advances our basic humanitarian values . . . support for global health has also proven its broader value in bolstering US national security and building constructive new partnerships . . . A smart, strategic long-term global health policy will advance America's core interests' (Fallon and Gayle 2010: 9). In a rather more overt example of how some leading US figures saw health contributing to foreign policy, former US Secretary of Health Tommy G. Thompson argues:

> [I]f we have any hope of spreading democracy and ending tyranny in every corner of the globe, it is vital that we use all of the weapons of freedom at our disposal. That includes our most effective arsenal against terrorists and the forces of oppression: education, compassion, and medicine. That is the principle at the heart of what I call 'medical diplomacy' – the winning of [the] hearts and minds of people in the Middle East, Asia, Africa, and elsewhere by exporting medical care, expertise, and personnel to help those who need it most. Medical diplomacy must be made a significantly larger part of our foreign and defense policy, as we clean up from costly and deadly wars in Afghanistan and Iraq. America has the best chance to win the war on terror and defeat the terrorists by enhancing our medical and humanitarian assistance to vulnerable countries. By delivering hope, we will deliver freedom. (Thompson 2005)

This is not to suggest that the sole motivation of providing health aid is to cyni-cally 'win friends and influence people'. Motivations in foreign policy tend to be more complex than this and the humanitarian impulse should not be dis-missed. But it is also clear that the potential of using health as a means of attracting states has been both recognized and exploited in foreign policy (see, e.g., Bonventre et al. 2009).

policy. Thus, debates may be about health rights versus trading interests, about free trade versus the protection of health services, or between the interests of the poor versus the privileged.

Security

The first two areas of intersection, security and governance, are among the most important issues to emerge in the development of a narrative on health and international relations and therefore are addressed in chapters of their own later in this book. They concern how foreign policy is used to protect the state and its citizens from health risks (security), and the institutional arrangements structuring the collective actions of state and non-state actors over health issues (governance). These two areas also share a common feature, namely the traditional (but increasingly contested) primacy of state-centric constructions: that is, that the state is the dominant actor involved. With security this construction is often termed 'national security', and is challenged at the intersection with health by other constructions which place either the individual at the centre of security (human security) or which are concerned with the promotion of health globally (global health security). Increased concern over the spread of disease, the potential use of biological weapons, and fears of health crises affecting the political stability and economic performance of weak states have contributed to health appearing on security agendas. This is discussed more fully in chapter 6, but the key points to note here are threefold. First, when foreign policy engages with health over security, it is primarily to promote and protect the state rather than the individual. The national security perspective therefore dominates over human security. This is not to say that concerns are not expressed over the health of individuals, but this is expressed in terms of the state's responsibility to its citizens. As Elbe (2009) and Ingram (2010) both note, this is a particular form of state power, which Foucault terms governmentality (see section on national and international security in chapter 6), and therefore remains locked into a state-centric rather than human-centric approach. The Institute of Medicine's 1997 report was therefore working from the basis of national security (governmentality), rather than human security, in arguing that '[t]he US government has a vital responsibility to protect all its citizens – its resident population, its soldiers and its travellers' (Institute of Medicine 1997: 4). Armitage and Nye's call for the US to redeem its image and influence abroad is premised on the use of 'smart power', including global health engagement, to achieve 'a more secure America' (2007: 1).

Second, as already described, the agenda from a foreign policy perspective has tended to be narrowly focused on a limited range of issues (see McInnes and Lee 2006). Although other issues have been raised, including more recently non-communicable diseases (NCDs), the focus has remained on severe and acute infectious disease outbreaks, bioterrorism and HIV/AIDS in terms of frequency of reference, priority accorded to them and resources allocated. And, as with the first point, these issues are generally constructed in a state-centric manner where the interests and responsibilities of the state predominate. Third, although there is clear potential for health and foreign policy to work together for mutual benefit, there are equally occasions where the interests of one pulls in a different direction from the other. In these instances, the interests of foreign policy in promoting national security have tended to prevail over those of health promotion. This is not to say that there are no humanitarian impulses in foreign policy, nor that policies such as foreign aid for health promotion is solely motivated by calculations of national interest and political benefit (*realpolitik*). But what does appear to be the case is that, when health and foreign policy overlap but pull in different directions, foreign policy appears to have greater sway with decision makers. In a paper for the US Council on Foreign Relations, for example, Jordan Kassalow is explicit in seeing engagement with global health issues as a tool for promoting US interests (including democracy promotion) *through* improving health: 'Supporting public health worldwide will enhance US national security, increase prosperity at home and abroad, promote democracy in developing countries and those in transition' (Kassalow 2001: 4; see also Feldbaum et al. 2010: 83–4). Similarly, the White House justified President Barack Obama's 2009 Global Health Initiative as 'an important component of the *national security* "smart power" strategy' (White House 2009, emphasis added). Even the UN somewhat despairingly pleaded that '[t]he increasing frequency with which global health issues and initiatives appear in all foreign policy contexts . . . must be understood to be more than a focus on specific diseases or an instrument of foreign policy' (UNGA 2010: 12).

Governance

Like security, governance has traditionally lent itself to state-centric constructions – that is, the manner in which states have cooperated for mutual benefit, sometimes allowing part of their sovereignty to be compromised either out of enlightened self-interest or for the greater good. The origins of international health cooperation in the nineteenth century lay in powerful states working together for their own mutual benefit. This pattern accorded with the so-called 'Westphalian' system, established by the 1648 Treaty of Westphalia which recognized a structure of independent sovereign states in Europe. The Westphalian system is 'anarchic', in the sense that there is no overarching governing power, although agreed rules and norms of behaviour exist which moderate the actions of states. Crucially for global health governance, there is agreement in this system to adopt certain health practices or protocols, including the international monitoring and surveillance of certain types of disease outbreaks. Such practices are not forced on states, except perhaps in extreme instances through the application of power by other states. Rather states choose to behave in accordance with international agreements or standards because they consider it in their best interests to do so.

More recent analyses have begun to suggest that the traditional Westphalian system of international health cooperation appears to be under threat from a variety of directions. At a normative level, concerns have been increasingly expressed that the globalization of health means that inter-state cooperation is no longer sufficient. What is required, it has been argued, are forms of global health governance which transcend individual state interests. At an organizational level, non-state players have become major actors in the global health policy arena. The World Bank, for example, began to view health as an important element in promoting economic development and growth in the 1980s. The view that poor health impeded development, and thus helped to keep poor states poor, led the substantially increased Bank lending for health development (Buse 1994). In contrast, the World Trade Organization (WTO) became involved in global health almost by accident through its attempts to globalize intellectual property rights. Because of the negative effect of the agreement on Trade-Related Intellectual Property Rights (TRIPS) on equitable access to medicines, especially anti-retroviral therapies for the treatment of HIV/AIDS, the WTO became the subject of furious campaigning by civil society organizations, patient groups and HIV/AIDS advocates, on the one hand, and pharmaceutical companies, on the other. The issue led to the adoption of the Doha Declaration on the TRIPS agreement and Public Health in 2001, reaffirming the flexibilities available to member states seeking to protect public health, followed by the Paragraph 6 Decision further clarifying the scope of these flexibilities (Sell 2003; Kerry and Lee 2007; Garrett 2007).

The international landscape also changed through the emergence of public-private partnerships, most notably those inspired by the Global Fund to Fight HIV/AIDS, Tuberculosis and Malaria agreed at the Group of Eight (G8) summit in Genoa in 2001. These partnerships, which combined public funds and private (often charitable), were particularly geared to developing new drugs and vaccines for those diseases traditionally neglected by the market-driven research and development (R&D) strategies of the pharmaceutical industry. But in so doing they acknowledged and contributed to the growing role and significance of charitable foundations in global health, especially the Bill and Melinda Gates Foundation, opening the door for greater policy influence. The WHO also sought to act in new ways, less as primarily a source of technical expertise and convenor of member states, and more as an independent actor in its own right. The WHO's issuance of travel advisories during the SARS outbreak of 2002–3, over the wishes of several governments, and the revision of the International Health Regulations (IHR 2005), appeared to give the organization new impetus to go beyond the reins of member states to, for example, obtain information on disease outbreaks of international concern.

These developments, in turn, posed crucial questions for the role of foreign policy in global health. At the heart was whether, to use Fidler's term, global health was moving to a 'post-Westphalian' system (Fidler 2003; Fidler and Gostin 2006) where anarchy was being replaced by a system of global health governance. If Fidler was correct in his observation that a revolution was taking place, then foreign policy was becoming less important in global health than the decisions of global actors such as the WHO. For the majority of global health watchers, however, the changes were interpreted as much less dramatic. While few would deny that new actors had appeared in force in global health policy making, and that established organizations had acquired new powers and roles, states equally appeared to be reinforced as the key actors, and foreign policy remained crucial in the manner in which they related to each other on health and other matters. As the Oslo Declaration put it: 'Often a public health threat in one country requires a concerted response that calls for many foreign policy makers to work together . . . The most effective response to global health challenges depends on alliances, cooperation, and partnerships that reflect a respect for national sovereignty and a sense of shared responsibility' (Oslo Declaration 2007: 1375).

Development

Foreign aid or overseas/official development assistance (ODA) is an occasionally uncomfortable bedfellow with foreign policy. Prompted by humanitarian impulses, aid programmes have bestowed significant benefits in the developing world, including addressing many health issues. Stuart Harris, for example, comments that:

> Humanitarian motives in foreign-aid policy were substantially behind past contributions by Australia to the world-wide eradication of smallpox and, particularly in our region, poliomyelitis, as well as to the successful training and support of skilled healthcare workers regionally. Furthermore, food aid from Australia supports global humanitarian efforts to limit morbidity and mortality from malnutrition. (Harris 2004: 172)

However, as Harris and others (e.g., Garrett 2007; Feldbaum et al. 2010) have pointed out, this humanitarianism generally co-exists with the promotion of national interests. Functionally foreign aid is often located within ministries of foreign affairs, and its priorities are influenced by the foreign policy interests of the donor states, especially as regards security and economic interests. But this tension between altruism and self-interest, between humanitarianism and *realpolitik*, is not simply a choice over who should receive aid. It can also be reflected less obviously in the type of aid given and, in the context of this book, what health issues are prioritized. The health development policies of the World Bank and the IMF provide an apt example. Critics (e.g., Colgan 2002) argue that both subordinated humanitarianism to the interests of major donors, as the main financiers of the two institutions, through the 'conditionalities' under which they made aid available to recipient countries during the 1980s and 1990s. These conditions, in short, privileged western market economies and their neo-liberal policy approaches. The economic crisis of the 1980s forced poor countries, especially in sub-Saharan Africa, to apply to the Bretton Woods institutions for temporary funding to stabilize their economies. Although this funding was provided, the conditions attached to this financing forced their governments to adopt economic development models and related policies that integrated these countries into the emerging world economy. Such policies included trade liberalization, privatization and cuts in public expenditure (including health services and financing). Subsequent evidence suggests these 'structural adjustments' resulted in states eventually repaying more (principal and interest) than in healthcare, particularly undermining the capacity of many countries to respond to the HIV/AIDS crisis in the late 1990s (Colgan 2002). By the late 1990s development policy appeared to be in crisis. The gap between rich and poor had grown, foreign aid contributions were in decline, structural adjustment had led to catastrophic levels of debt, and in Africa the HIV crisis was in full swing. Gro Harlem Brundtland was frank in her assessment that 'the war on poverty has failed' (Brundtland 1999: 3).

However, the new millennium proved something of a turning point. Levels of foreign aid and the political priority given to development both increased substantially, not least by the G8 (see box 3.3), but also by a proliferation of new global health actors and initiatives (McCoy et al. 2009). In the US in particular, foreign aid increased including US$15 billion committed over five years for HIV/AIDS under the US President's Emergency Plan for AIDS Relief (PEPFAR). Most notably, in September 2000 at the Millennium Summit, world leaders agreed to the MDGs, with the aim of reducing poverty by half alongside a range of other identified goals by 2015 (see box 3.4). Significantly, health featured prominently in the MDGs, reflecting a new consensus that, although many suffered ill-health because of poverty, many were also poor because they were sick (e.g., Institute of Medicine 1997: 2; Colgan 2002; Labonte 2004: 160). Investing in health therefore appeared to be, not only an important humanitarian gesture to improve health, but also a sensible investment for economic development. Von Schirnding, for example, noted, 'Malaria . . . has slowed economic growth in endemic countries in Africa by up to 1.3 per cent per year. Africa's gross domestic product would probably be about US$100 billion higher if malaria had been tackled 30 years ago when effective control measures first became available' (Von Schirnding 2002: 633). Towards the end of the decade, a US intelligence community assessment for the National Intelligence Council (NIC) was able to conclude:

> considerable empirical and theoretical studies have been done on the relationship between health and *economic* growth and development. The clearest evidence of a causal link has been the economic impact of high-profile infectious diseases. Historically, progress on health issues has correlated in a number of countries with improved economic development and growth by expanding the pool of healthy and productive workers . . . attention to health issues is a key determinant as to whether countries can escape poverty. (NIC 2008: 23)

The NIC report drew specific attention to SARS which 'caused a significant, if temporary, slowing of economic growth in East Asia and Canada' and HIV/AIDS and malaria in sub-Saharan Africa which 'dampened' economic growth (NIC 2008: 23). This contrasted with improvements to health achieved in Mexico and Singapore through investments in health care infrastructure and disease control which, in turn, had led to economic growth and poverty reduction. The narrative reflected in the NIC report was clear: investing in health makes economic sense with both local and global benefits in terms of poverty reduction and economic growth. Although the global economic crisis which began in 2008 appears to threaten this new level of funding, Stuckler et al.

Box 3.3 The Group of Eight countries and ODA

At its Gleneagles summit in 2005, the G8 committed to doubling its ODA to Africa by 2010 to $50 billion a year (Gleneagles Communiqué 2005). Prior to its Deauville Summit in 2011, the G8 released an *Accountability Report* detailing how it had responded to its Gleneagles commitments. The report stated:

> During the 2005 G8 Gleneagles Summit, G8 Leaders and other donors announced a range of commitments on increasing Official Development Assistance. Each G8 country made specific commitments to increase ODA . . . Since 2004, the G8 has accounted for nearly 70% of total ODA from all OECD-DAC donors and its ODA contributions have increased by more than 54%. During this period, the G8 increased its ODA by $31.2 billion while the global ODA from all OECD-DAC donors has increased by more than $48 billion. Despite budgetary constraints, the G8 has maintained its fiscal efforts with an ODA increase of $7.3 billion between 2009 and 2010. This increase represents 82% of the overall increase from DAC donors of $8.9 billion between 2009 and 2010. While recognizing that not all our Gleneagles commitments were met and that a gap in financing for development remains, the G8 flags the sharp increase in ODA since 2004, as well as the results obtained and the progress accomplished in the way of delivering ODA. (G8 2011)

However aid agencies such as Oxfam were more critical:

> The commitment, made at Gleneagles in 2005 after the high-profile Make Poverty History campaign, was for rich countries to provide an extra £30 billion of international aid by 2010. However the figures for the year, released today by the Organization for Economic Cooperation and Development (OECD), show a massive shortfall of £11 billion. (Oxfam 2011)

Although the OECD noted that in 2010 aid flows from DAC donor countries were the highest ever and represented a 6.5% increase over 2009, it also noted that Africa was likely to receive less than half of the increase the G8 had committed themselves to at Gleneagles, 'mainly a result of the underperformance of some European donors' (OECD, 2012).

(2011c) argue that there is no statistically significant evidence of a relationship between past recessions and levels of health aid disbursed by states (although whether the same applies to private foundations, which may find their income affected from poor returns on investments, is not examined).

The increased funding and political attention from the G8 and others for development in general, and health in particular, has not been without criticism. Some questions raised are generic to ODA: whether aid commitments have been matched with disbursements, whether excessive amounts of money are being siphoned off (legally or illegally)

Box 3.4 The Millennium Development Goals

The MDGs were agreed by world leaders at the UN in September 2000, with a series of targets to be reached by 2015. The eight headline goals were:

1. To eradicate extreme poverty and hunger.
2. To achieve universal primary education.
3. To promote gender equality and empower women.
4. To reduce child mortality.
5. To improve maternal health.
6. To combat HIV/AIDS, malaria and other major diseases.
7. To ensure environmental sustainability.
8. To develop a global partnership for development.

Each of these goals had a series of more detailed targets, with a timeframe building up to 2015.

Source: UN (no date)

before they reach those in need, and whether the multiple donors involved could organize their efforts more efficiently and effectively (for examples of these general concerns applied to health, see Garrett 2007 and McCoy et al. 2009). But two related concerns raised about health development aid are particularly interesting. The first is the manner in which aid is 'stove piped' into narrow programmes or disease-specific treatments; and the second is whether aid is related to need. What underpins both of these is a critique that ODA for health reflects the interests of the donors as much – and perhaps sometimes more – than the needs of recipients. Despite PEPFAR providing millions of Africans with access to anti-retroviral treatment for the first time, for example, US HIV prevention policy in Africa under the George W. Bush administration advocated abstinence and fidelity, rather than the use of condoms and needle exchange, reflecting the administration's moral stance rather than the advice of health workers in Africa. A study by Oomman et al. (2007: 18–19) also suggests that PEPFAR funding policy, rather than the specific needs of Mozambique, Uganda and Zambia, have taken precedent, observing that 'the similarity of funding allocations is striking given the epidemiological differences among these three countries' (see figure 3.1). Jeremy Youde (2010b) demonstrates that funding for HIV/AIDS does not necessarily go to the states with highest prevalence but reflects other strategic priorities. Moreover, the relatively large increase in funding for HIV/AIDS also reflected donors' interest in that particular disease over others. In 1998, HIV accounted for 5 per cent of ODA for health, but by 2007 this had increased to 47 per cent, during a period when the ODA budget for health itself

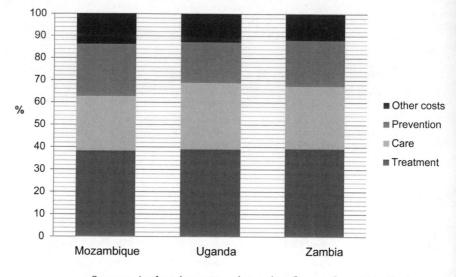

Source: Authors' construction using figures from http://www. pepfar.org.

Figure 3.1 *PEPFAR fiscal year 2007 approved funding by programme area and country*

expanded enormously (Moran et al. 2008; Feldbaum et al. 2010: 84). Although there is no doubt that HIV/AIDS represents one of the major health challenges of contemporary times, and requires considerably more funding than has so far been provided, other health conditions which account for millions more deaths annually remain comparatively underfunded. A 'hierarchy' of diseases can therefore be identified, in terms of funding priority, for which need is but one consideration. As Feldbaum et al. (2010: 84) comment, 'foreign policy's powerful influence on development assistance for health leaves many pressing global health battles under resourced but allows global health efforts that do align with foreign policy interests to receive significant political support and funding'.

Human rights

The idea of a human right to health has a long and distinguished history (Evans 2002: 197; see also box 3.5). Establishing this right at an international level is a more recent phenomenon, but nevertheless has been achieved not least through a series of declarations, including the WHO Constitution and Declaration of the 1978 International Conference on Primary Health Care at Alma Ata (see box 3.6), as well the Universal Declaration of Human Rights and the UN International Convention on Economic, Social and Cultural Rights. The latter establishes both an obligation on states to provide a minimum set of health services and outlines means of realizing them. Moreover, although most international human rights agreements focus on individuals, rather than the population level focus of public health, the 1986 UN Declaration on the Right to Development does locate the right to health at the community level. Despite the above declarations, Labonte and Gagnon note that the right to health is poorly located in the actual international human rights framework which remains heavily centred on the rights of the individual (Labonte 2004: 159–60; Labonte and Gagnon 2010: 11).

Human rights and the right to health also feature prominently in many of the statements which link foreign policy and health, often

---

Box 3.5 The human right to health

The human right to the highest attainable standard of health has both a legal and normative basis. The legal basis derives from a range of international treaties and declarations, many of which have been developed over the period since the end of the Second World War, and national constitutions, over a hundred of which guarantee a right to health (Hunt 2006; Susser 1993; Leary 1994). The normative basis often manifests itself as a sense of despair at the suffering of others but is motivated by concepts of social justice (e.g., Pogge 2005). Both acknowledge that this is a 'work in progress', with resource limits and a lack of will being the two most commonly identified reasons for the failure to achieve universal implementation.

As Toebes points out, 'in . . . international human rights, economic, social, and cultural rights are generally distinguished from civil and political rights' (Toebes 1999: 661). This derives from the distinction between what are often called 'positive' and 'negative' rights. Civil and political rights tend to be negative – the argument being that government and society should not interfere in certain areas of life, for example freedom of speech or of association. Positive rights, however, require action to change, improve or protect an area of life. The human right to health is therefore a positive right in that it requires action on the part of government and society to secure it. But the problem here is the manner in which rights have been constructed. In what Tony Evans has described as the dominant 'liberal consensus', whereas negative rights should be guaranteed internationally, positive rights should only be treated as 'aspirations' because of the resource implications involved (Evans, 2002). Thus commentators such as Barlow can comment that 'it is difficult to find any rational or utilitarian basis for viewing health care in the same way [as civil and political rights]' (cited in Evans 2002: 197). But as is demonstrated in the work of critics such as Pogge and Evans, this need not be so; rather it is a choice which privileges some issues and interests over others.

claiming the right to health as 'fundamental', and sometimes claiming this as the driving force behind this link (see, e.g., Labonte and Gagnon 2010: 11–12). It is also highlighted in a number of foreign policy statements including the Oslo Declaration, which explicitly based itself on 'the recognition that life is the most fundamental of human rights, and that life and health are the most precious assets' (Oslo Declaration 2007: 1374). The international focus on health as a right has also been seen in developments such as the appointment of a special rapporteur on health by the UN Commissioner for Human Rights, and the attention given to it by the Human Rights Council (Labonte 2004: 159–60; UNGA 2010: 9).

Despite this, and despite the WHO's use of health as a human right in various campaigns in the first few decades after its establishment, the health rights agenda gained little political purchase beyond the public health field. Indeed, even in development policy, health assis-

Box 3.6 The Alma Ata Declaration

The 1978 International Conference on Primary Health Care, held at Alma-Ata in modern day Kazakhstan, provided the catalyst for the WHO's 'Health for All' policy. This policy was based on the twin ideas that primary health care constituted a human right and that health should be a key element of development strategies aimed at tackling social and economic inequalities. The Alma Ata Declaration stated:

[Health] is a fundamental human right and that the attainment of the highest possible level of health is a most important world-wide social goal whose realization requires the action of many other social and economic sectors in addition to the health sector.

The existing gross inequality in the health status of the people particularly between developed and developing countries as well as within countries is politically, socially and economically unacceptable and is, therefore, of common concern to all countries . . . The promotion and protection of the health of the people is essential to sustained economic and social development and contributes to a better quality of life and to world peace. The people have the right and duty to participate individually and collectively in the planning and implementation of their health care. Governments have a responsibility for the health of their people which can be fulfilled only by the provision of adequate health and social measures. A main social target of governments, international organizations and the whole world community in the coming decades should be the attainment by all peoples of the world by the year 2000 of a level of health that will permit them to lead a socially and economically productive life. Primary health care is the key to attaining this target as part of development in the spirit of social justice. (WHO 1978)

tance tended to be promoted as a means out of poverty, rather than as a human right in itself. This began to change, however, for a number of reasons. Among these, globalization appears to have been a facilitating condition rather than a primary driver. It established a context whereby health was seen in global terms, and by association rights to health were equally seen in these terms, although as London and Schneider (2011) point out, globalization also threatened the right to health by disempowering states. Much more important was the work of activists and practitioners working in the field of HIV/AIDS. These individuals and their associated organizations promoted international action on the disease, not through a public health route (for example, by trying to amend the existing International Health Regulations to include HIV), but through a rights-based framework. The rights of people living with HIV/AIDS were emphasized not just as a means of dealing with the stigma associated with the disease in many societies, but as a means of encouraging international action to prevent the spread of, and assisting those living with, the disease.

Three examples highlight the manner in which the rights agenda has come up against other foreign policy agendas in relation to HIV/AIDS. The first concerns the campaign to amend the TRIPS agreement which, by upholding patent protection worldwide, hindered the sale of affordable generic anti-retroviral therapies produced by drug companies who did not hold the patent rights. In this example, industry interests in protecting the considerable R&D investment required to bring new drugs to market through patent rights were opposed by arguments maintaining the rights of people living with HIV/AIDS, many of whom live in the world's poorest countries, to have access to medicines critical to prolonging their lives (see also section below on international trade). Second, AIDS activists successfully challenged a government policy in South Africa which prevented people diagnosed as HIV positive from serving in the armed forces. The South African military were concerned about the operational and cost implications for national security, while HIV/AIDS activists complained that this was discriminatory and infringed the rights of individuals (Heinecken 2003). A similar law was introduced through the US Congress in the 1990s on national security grounds, but was quickly withdrawn with President Bill Clinton framing his own objections clearly using rights-based terms, describing the law as 'unconstitutional, completely abhorrent and offensive' (quoted in Sjostedt 2010: 158). Finally, a number of countries have attempted to prevent people diagnosed as HIV positive from entering as immigrants (see, e.g., Bisaillon 2010). In 1993, for example, the Clinton administration detained 270 Haitian political refugees seeking asylum at

Guantanamo because of concerns that high HIV prevalence in their home country would impact on US national security (Sjostedt 2010: 158).

The issue of health rights is by no means limited to HIV/AIDS. It featured prominently during the SARS outbreak when mandatory quarantine and isolation measures were used to control the spread of the disease (Farmer and Campos 2007), and has similarly been raised with reference to access to anti-viral drugs and vaccines in pandemic influenza preparedness policies (Kamradt-Scott and Lee, forthcoming). As well as human rights clashing with other foreign policy interests, the issues point to tensions between two separate rights – the right of individuals to free movement and association, and the collective right to health of societies as expressed by measures to prevent and control the spread of disease outbreaks. Historically, public health practice has privileged collective over individual rights, with the suspension of the latter in order to protect the community at large. One of the most dramatic examples of this is the belief that hundreds of residents of Mary King's Close in the Old Town of Edinburgh were bricked up alive during the seventeenth century, following an outbreak of bubonic plague, for fear that the contagion would spread to other parts of the city. While contemporary public health practice has since progressed dramatically, the delicate balance between individual and collective rights can be observed in the legal frameworks adopted by each country regulating public health risks, notably when non-cooperation by individuals is encountered (see, e.g., the UK Health Protection Regulations 2010 and Hong Kong Prevention and Control of Disease Ordinance 2011). How such regulations seek to control the cross/transborder spread of diseases, potentially infringing on individual rights when deemed necessary, and possibly creating spillover effects on domestic and foreign economies, gives such actions foreign policy dimensions. The revised International Health Regulations (2005) requires member states to protect the dignity and rights of travellers when applying disease control measures (Fidler 2010: 8).

Beyond infectious disease outbreaks, the rights-based agenda has been extended to such issues as maternal and child health (MCH) and the migration of health care workers. The first of these is important because it indicates a broadening of interest in the health and foreign policy arena to a wider spectrum of health conditions and vulnerable populations (UNGA 2010: 9; Sridhar et al. 2011; UNGA 2011). The second reveals two tensions concerning health, human rights and foreign policy – between the right of freedom of movement and the right to health; and between the promotion of trade interests, especially the promotion of free trade, and the promotion and protection of rights. At its heart is the concern that health professionals will be distributed according to wealth of populations and not health need. Kanchanachitra et al. (2011) note, for example, how free movement has led to the maldistribution of health workers in Southeast Asia. The global imbalance of health workers is stark, especially between sub-Saharan African countries and high-income countries in the US and Europe. As Anyangwe and Mtonga describe,

> About 59 million people make up the health workforce of paid full-time health workers world-wide . . . The Americas (mainly USA and Canada) are home to 14% of the world's population, bear only 10% of the world's disease burden, have 37% of the global health workforce and spend about 50% of the world's financial resources for health. Conversely, sub-Saharan Africa, with about 11% of the world's population bears over 24% of the global disease burden, is home to only 3% of the global health workforce, and spends less than 1% of the world's financial resources on health. (Anyangwe and Mtonga 2007: 93).

These imbalances, fuelled by the active recruitment of health care workers from poor regions, has led to the adoption of a number of voluntary codes and agreements including a 2010 WHO Global Code of Practice on the International Recruitment of Health Personnel (e.g., Dhillon et al. 2010; Plotnikova 2011). These agreements, however, remain 'soft law' given their lack of binding authority, weak enforcement mechanisms, and reliance on good will and voluntary compliance in their implementation.

International Trade

In contemporary foreign policy narratives, the growth of international trade is framed positively and unproblematically, by the Bretton Woods institutions, G8, World Economic Forum, OECD member states and most UN bodies, as promoting economic growth nationally and globally (Rose 2005). The development and promotion of trade liberalization is thus accepted as a core foreign policy objective. The growth in international trade since the end of the Second World War, is also seen as one of the key drivers behind globalization, the spread of which underpins, in turn, many of the linkages drawn between global health and International Relations identified in this book. The relationship between trade and health, however, has proved to be both a source of friction and cooperation. As mentioned at the beginning of this chapter, trade can facilitate the spread of disease through the increased crossborder movement of people, goods and services. Trade liberalization can also create other direct risks to health, such as enabling the growth in health-harming substances such as tobacco, guns and hazardous materials. Or it can cause indirect harms to health by leading to a world economy supplied, in part at least, by production chains underpinned by poor quality and weakly regulated working and living conditions (Loewenson 2001). At the same time, a growth in international trade can lead to improved health by the creation of gainful employment, downward pressures on prices, and increased availability of health-promoting goods and services such as fresh fruits and vegetables (Flanagan 2006).

The balancing of economic costs and benefits of trade, with the costs and benefits to health, has challenged international health cooperation, from the International Sanitary Conventions of the nineteenth century, to more contemporary agreements such as the FCTC (2003), IHR (2005) and Pandemic Influenza Preparedness Framework (2011). Powerful industry interests have sought to play major roles in the development of such agreements (see, e.g., Collin et al. 2002), and the comparatively small number of accords suggests the enduring power of these lobbies. Developing effective regulation at the national level has proved similarly problematic. It is reported that effective and full implementation of the FCTC at country level has been undermined by industry interests in Argentina (Mejia et al. 2008), China (Wan et al. 2011), Germany (Grüning et al. 2011) and many other countries. The series of food-related events over the past two decades, including bovine spongiform encephalopathy (BSE) and variant Creutzfeldt-Jakob disease (or so-called mad cow disease), melamine-contaminated milk products in China, and fears of contamination of food supplies from damaged nuclear power plants following the Japanese earthquake and tsunami of 2011, without a strong regulatory response internationally suggests another realm where trade interests continue to prevail (Lin 2011).

In a further twist to this relationship, agreements to promote trade can create health risks. The most commonly cited example of this is the TRIPS agreement to protect international patent (IP) rights. In requiring all WTO members to adopt Western-style protection for patents the agreement threatened the availability of cheap drugs to the poorest countries. Although Pauwelyn (2010) suggests TRIPS was an agreement with more bark than bite, especially after the Doha round introduced new flexibilities to the agreement under pressure from public health interests, others such as Aginam (2010) argue that the system still disadvantages the poorest states and impedes access to essential medicines. That both trade interests and public health remain unhappy over TRIPS and IP, despite Doha, reveals that there remain unresolved tensions. In a similar vein, some health specialists (e.g., Pollock and Price, 2000; Labonte, 2004: 161) have expressed concern over the potential impact on health services of the General Agreement on Tariffs and Trade (GATT) Treaty, which attempted to open up public services to competition on international markets. As with TRIPS, the fear was that public health, especially for the poorest, would suffer as a result of trading interests. The tensions over GATTS and TRIPS both reflected the fact that health had become big business, with hundreds of billions of dollars being spent on health care globally each year. The international political economy of health is discussed later in this book (see chapter 4), but for this chapter the key point this raises is that, for some power-ful states, health is an important industry which needs to be protected and promoted internationally _as a business_.

Health crises can, of course, disrupt trade significantly. In the UK, the BSE crisis in the 1990s, and the 2002 foot and mouth outbreak, both led to restrictions on the trade of certain British meat products. Similarly, the SARS outbreak led to a substantial reduction in travel to the Asian region, and the 2011 outbreak of _E. coli_ in Germany led Russia to suspend the import of food stuffs from the European Union. Moreover the perception of illness can lead to bans on the trade of goods uncon-nected to the outbreak. Conversely, the argument that investing in health can create better markets for goods and services has also received considerable attention. The US Institute of Medicine (1997: 9) argued that 'healthier populations abroad would also constitute more vibrant markets for US goods and services', a theme reflected two years later by WHO Director-General Gro Harlem Brundtland (1999: 3) and in the WHO's Commission on Macroeconomics and Health (WHO 2001).

The relationship between health and foreign policy nevertheless is most often characterized as one of risk to health from increased trade, with foreign policy interests often being more closely aligned with the former than the latter. This is what underpins the Oslo Declaration's plea that 'international trade policies and agreements need to be placed within the context of protecting and promoting well being' (Oslo Declaration 2007: 1378). In a slightly more optimistic vein, the UN Secretary General's _Note_ to the 2010 UN General Assembly Special Session on global health and foreign policy argued that, 'in these dynamics of interdependence, health is no longer automatically subject to other interests, but other policies may have to adjust in order to meet the health prerogative' (UNGA 2010: 6). The _Note_ proceeds to identify a series of agreements where trade interests have been moderated to accommodate those of health. We seem however to be still some way from a relationship where cooperation is the norm; rather the relationship appears to be one largely driven by trade interests, whether in protecting trade or developing new markets, occasionally moderated by cooperative agreements to protect health.

Global Public Goods for Health

Economists have long understood the idea of public goods, namely that certain desirable goods or services must be provided through public intervention because of market failure (i.e. the private sector lacks the necessary incentives). Thus peace and security is in the interests of those who live and work within a state, but in the modern age is provided for by the state (public intervention) through its security policy because, although private industries benefit from the stability this might provide, none has sufficient incentive and/or capacity to provide it by itself. 'Global public goods' however is a more recent development, a concept which recognizes that this same logic can be applied across borders – that there may be global benefits from some developments, but that it is not sufficiently in any one state's interest or capacity to undertake these developments alone. Instead cooperation is required, not just between states and traditional international institutions, but potentially with non-state actors such as civil society organizations and private-public partnerships. The corollary is that 'global public bads', such as unstable climate change and disease outbreaks, are characterized by a lack of cooperation leading to collective difficulties. 'Global public goods for health' is more recent still, being largely a twenty-first-century idea. It is often linked to the requirement for some form of global health governance or global health diplomacy to ensure that these are delivered. The application of global public goods theory to health is most often seen when dealing with policies for infectious disease control, especially pandemics (Labonte and Gagnol 2010: 7). The surveillance of disease outbreaks, measures taken for their containment and the development of effective interventions transcend national interests and serve the global interest, warranting initiatives such as the Global Outbreak Alert and Response Network (GOARN), funding of vaccine programmes and initiatives to tackle neglected diseases. Moreover weakness at the national level may mean that one state's lack of preparedness creates a risk globally. Concerns over the capacity of low- to middle-income countries to prepare for an influenza pandemic, for example, is compounded by fears that some of these countries are among the most likely to be the geographical source of a new virus. Thus, cooperation may require more than coordination but active assistance, facilitated by global health governance and/or diplomacy. This assistance may involve technical assistance such as strengthening the capacity to undertake surveillance to provide early warning of disease outbreaks, collecting samples and identifying a disease; it might involve stockpiling vaccines and other drugs in advance of an outbreak as part of a strategy to prevent it spreading more widely; or, more ambitiously, it may involve preventative measures such as health system strengthening and addressing up-stream causes of ill-health (e.g., poor sanitation and housing). At an even more macro level, it may involve international regulation of health-harming products or practices, whether industrial (nuclear, chemical, biological or radiological) or foodstuffs including tobacco and foods with a high sugar/fat/salt content.

SARS provides an excellent example of this: information on the spread of the disease, the means by which people became infected, the identification of the disease as a new form of the corona virus, and the development of vaccines, was widely portrayed as a global effort because shared interests were at stake. One narrative of the SARS crisis, therefore, constructed it as an example of how the world could – and should – work cooperatively together for mutual benefit. Similarly post-SARS pandemic influenza preparedness is depicted in many narratives, not as a national concern, but as a global effort justifying global resources in terms of surveillance, monitoring and virus sharing. For some, the emergence of global public goods for health implies the need for, and even the beginnings of a movement towards, a new political relationship where global governance of health issues feature prominently, not least in disease surveillance, and one which extends far beyond technical cooperation and the exchange of scientific data. For these, the actions of WHO during the SARS outbreak, where the organization appeared to act in the collective interest beyond the self-interest of individual states, and the manner in which negotiations on the revised IHRs were more quickly concluded after SARS, when previously they had stalled, indicates how fear spurred the rapid development of the new relationship between health and foreign policy.

This narrative, with its strong normative dimension of promoting a 'global commons', almost certainly overstates the long-term political significance of events such as WHO's response to SARS. A different construction of what happened is possible, however, based on enlightened national self-interests, which may also explain the emergence of interest in global public goods for health. In this construction, states cooperate even when the returns are not immediately obvious, because of the realization that *at some point* the process of cooperation will benefit them. Labonte (2004: 160–1) suggests global public goods for health is less about the shift away from a Westphalian system of self-help for states and towards global health governance, and more about a move-ment to broaden national interests in global health away from a focus on clear and present dangers. Thus, with SARS states cooperated because it was in their interests to do so lest the disease proved to be more dangerous and spread more widely than it did. The IHRs similarly gave member states a mechanism to deliver early warning of disease out-breaks emerging elsewhere and monitor their progress. Perhaps the most interesting example of interests and global public goods for health concerns Indonesia and virus sharing (see box 3.7). This revealed the extent to which an issue which could be presented as a clear example of a global public good for health, namely the sharing of data on and samples of new viruses, was also intimately bound up with the interests of the powerful.

Box 3.7 Indonesia and virus sharing

In 1952 WHO established the Global Influenza Virus Sharing Network (GISN) to identify new strains of the influenza virus and allow the development of new vaccines. The Network also acts as an alert mechanism, warning of novel strains which have the potential to become pandemic. Central to GISN is the manner in which samples of the influenza virus are passed on a systematic and regular basis from National Influenza Centres to one of six WHO Collaborating Centres worldwide. Here they are analysed, at no cost to the states submitting them, to determine which strains are in active circulation arising from minor changes to a virus (antigenic drift) and whether a new strain may be emerging from a major change to an influenza virus (antigenic shift). The distinction between the two enables planning for seasonal and potentially pandemic influenza. From this analysis WHO recommends the vaccines for circulating strains of influenza which, for seasonal influenza, results in the annual production of approximately 250 million doses of vaccine. GISN therefore appears to be an example of a global public good for health.

In early 2007, however, Indonesia decided to cease sharing its samples of the H5N1 influenza virus with WHO. This was especially serious since it came at a time when fears of a highly pathogenic influenza pandemic from this virus were high. Indonesia's Minister of Health, Siti Fadilah Supari, was central to this deci-sion, arguing that these virus samples were being passed on, without Indonesia's knowledge or permission, to private pharmaceutical companies to develop vac-cines. These vaccines were highly lucrative to the companies involved, with the price set being beyond the reach of most Indonesians and people in other Asian countries. At the same time, the region was more likely to be at the front line of an influenza pandemic. Moreover, patents had been taken out on the avian influenza virus, and Material Transfer Agreements were agreed between WHO and pharmaceutical companies without the consent of countries providing virus samples. Supari claimed that this practice was unfair and exploitative, a position shared by a number of other low- and middle-income countries. Indonesia's fears appeared vindicated in 2009–10 when, during the H1N1 (swine flu) pandemic, high-income countries had privileged access to vaccines through prior pre-purchasing agreements with manufacturers. There was little or no spare production capacity for populations in other countries, meaning that vaccines were available only to the governments of those countries, regardless of who was most at risk from an influenza pandemic and which governments had provided virus samples to manufacture the vaccines.

Although Indonesia's position was supported by a number of low- and middle-income countries, the general reaction, especially from the United States, was extremely hostile. At a time of world concern over the potential of an influenza pandemic, Indonesia's actions were criticized as reckless and threatening to global health security. The dispute rumbled on until April 2011 when the Pandemic Influenza Preparedness Framework was brokered by WHO. Under this agreement, virus sharing would continue and vaccine manufacturers would set aside at least 10 per cent of their production during a pandemic for low- and middle-income countries, at low or no cost. Additional measures were agreed to support such countries in the establishment of their own vaccine manufacturing capacity.

Sources: WHO (no date); WHO (2007d); Fidler (2008); Sinha (2011); Knox (2011); Kamradt-Scott and Lee (forthcoming).

Conclusion

This chapter examines how the relationship between health and foreign policy is constructed along six intersections. Some of these have achieved greater prominence than others, for example, security and governance compared to human rights and global public goods for health. This is not because, in some objective sense, these are more important. Rather the debate is constructed with these issues being important because that is what those who shape the debate believe or want it to be. Within these intersections, some health issues appear with regularity, especially infectious disease outbreaks in general, and SARS, pandemic influenza and HIV/AIDS in particular. Although the successful negotiation of the FCTC may be portrayed as an early example of the two communities working effectively together on a non-communicable disease area, it was only near the end of the first decade of the twenty-first century that NCDs began to be cited more prominently as important issues on the global health agenda. Doubts remain over the longevity of these issues beyond the 2011 UN General Assembly's High Level Meeting on NCDs. Nor are issues concerning a gamut of other health conditions affected by globalization significant on the contemporary global health and foreign policy agenda, despite considerable evidence to suggest they should be otherwise.

The narrative concerning the relationship between foreign policy and global health is fairly well-established: that it has its roots in international health cooperation in the nineteenth century; that for most of the twentieth century this relationship fell into abeyance, not least because foreign policy was focused on the high politics of power and security rather than the low politics of quality of life, but also because health policy focused on technocratic rather than political solutions to health problems; and that at the end of the century this relationship was re-established, not least because of the impact of globalization, culminating towards the end of the first decades in ideas of global health diplomacy. Underpinning much of this, from a public health perspective, is a normative agenda concerning how to create a healthier world. Although foreign policy reveals a normative dimension as well, in the sense of a commitment to humanitarianism, it is also motivated by interests, especially those involving trade and security.

Importantly, this narrative is not an independent objective assessment of a developing relationship, but a particular construction of part of the social world relating to global health which has established certain pathways for action. The power of the narrative is perhaps best seen in the relative lack of criticism over the central idea that, in an age of increased globalization, health and foreign policy need to work more closely together. But fewer still have questioned what work this narrative has done for global health. The dominant narrative is of two policy communities coming together out of shared interests across a variety of fields (identified here as the six intersections). This narrative has perpetuated a state-centric perspective, albeit one moderated by other 'new' actors, thereby creating the view that it is states that matter – their interests, actions and capabilities are key to global health. It has also allowed the development of a binary: that there are two separate communities whose interests overlap but may at times pull in different directions, and that the way to understand some of the tensions in global health is to understand the different interests and priorities of health and foreign policy. This binary not only limits the establishment of global health diplomacy as a single policy arena, but also suggests who the key players are in global health diplomacy and how to identify the key issues and intersections.

But other narratives are possible concerning the international relations of global health: narratives of the healthy and the suffering; narratives of rich and poor; and narratives of who owns and produces what in global health. The dominant narrative suggests that the coming together between health and foreign policy was something self-evident because globalization created a need for the two to work together. From a constructivist position, however, we are sceptical of relationships in the social world being portrayed as 'natural', since this often obscures rather than reveals what is really going on. Global health diplomacy, therefore, is not the 'natural' outcome of a process of cooperation prompted by globalization, but a way of constructing the world and establishing a type of outcomes which privileged certain ideas, interests and institutions over others.

CHAPTER FOUR

Global Health and the International Political Economy

In the broadest sense, political economy is concerned with the mutual shaping of the political and economic spheres. Since the 1970s, international political economy (IPE) has thrived as a rich and varied interdisciplinary field of study in International Relations, giving rise to robust and vigorous scholarly debate, about its nature and consequences. This chapter argues that global health, as a subject of scholarly and policy concern, can be more fully explained by locating it within the shifting balance between states and markets, the rise of transnational actors, and the consequent delineation of authority and responsibility. Correspondingly, our understanding of the IPE can benefit from a fuller understanding of global health, a realm which exemplifies the close interplay between the public and private spheres, as well as changes to structure and agency characterizing globalization. Key to this chapter is the idea that the blurring of the political and economic spheres is particularly evident in the emergence and social construction of global health as a concept and practice. This has led to major tensions between competing narratives on what global health is; how it should be produced and consumed within an increasingly global context; what knowledge should be discovered and how it should be used in global health; and how health equity is affected by the IPE. One dominant narrative, for example, is that the globalization of health care is a progressive development, underpinned by the desirability of liberalizing the 'markets' for health care services and financing, rationalizing health care production and consumption, and making more efficient use of increasingly scarce resources. However, as this chapter demonstrates, such arguments can be located within the IPE of global health, which prioritizes certain health conditions that are of concern to some, but not all, and is shaped by the transnational distribution of economic and political power. What we argue in this chapter is that a particular narrative of IPE has been dominant in global health. This narrative finds its origins in the neo-liberal economics of the 1980s and, although

modified and subject to evolution since then, the underpinning normative and theoretical basis remains constant. This narrative frames health
provision as an economic issue and focuses on the efficient allocation
of resources, rather than on the allocation of these resources for social
justice or other ends. Although it would be a mistake to interpret this
as a championing of an unrestricted free market in health, the clear
priority remains economic concerns with the public provision of health
services and care acting as a safety net or moderating force while private
industry and market mechanisms remain the dominant means of
ensuring efficiency.

Conceptualizing the International Political Economy of Global Health

In the 1970s, International Relations scholars drew renewed attention
to the need to understand the shifting balance between states (political
authority) and markets (economic relations). This led to a flourishing
of new thinking on the conceptualization of international political
economy (traditionally divided into liberal, nationalist and Marxist perspectives), the close relationship between economic and political power,
and the implications for a broad range of policy issues (Gilpin 1987).
Susan Strange, for example, wrote that 'It is impossible to have political
power without the power to purchase, to command production, to
mobilize capital. And it is impossible to have economic power without
the sanction of political authority' (Strange 1998: 25). In a world of
corporate behemoths, economic actors had become political actors.
Moreover, the large size of the state sector means that governments can
sometimes assert as much economic power as corporate actors in the
world economy. For IPE scholars, this mutual interdependence of powerful states and firms has defined and driven the trajectory of globalization over the past thirty years (Stopford and Strange 1991).

The aim of this chapter is to explore how IPE can extend our understanding of the narratives underpinning global health. The analysis of
global health from an IPE perspective has been limited to date. Lesley
Doyal's *The Political Economy of Health* provides an early account of the
structural factors that underpin 'the social production of health and
illness in capitalist societies', focusing on the UK and East Africa (Doyal
1979: 23). Vicente Navarro's work is also strongly informed by Marxist-
based approaches, explaining health inequalities within and across
national settings in terms of the spread of neo-liberal-based market
capitalism (Navarro 1982; Navarro and Muntaner 2004). These are
important critical analyses of how structural conditions shape health

outcomes, although they fall short of explaining how power within the IPE is expressed through competing narratives in global health.

Strange's distinction between relational and structural power is useful in this respect. *Relational power* is the power of A to get B to do what it would not otherwise do. *Structural power*, in contrast, 'confers the power to decide how things shall be done, the power to shape frameworks within which states relate to each other, relate to people, or relate to corporate enterprises' (Strange 1998: 25). She identifies four key interrelated structures underpinning the IPE: production, finance, knowledge and security. The *production structure* concerns who produces what, where, under what conditions, and how it is sold, to whom, and on what terms. The *financial structure* concerns the international monetary system and international finance and debt. The *knowledge structure* is about who has access to knowledge and technology, and on what terms. Finally, 'the *security structure* is the framework of power created by the provision of security by some human beings for others' (Strange 1998: 45). Other prominent IPE scholars, such as Robert Keohane and Joseph Nye, also challenged International Relation's state-centrism, arguing that the growth of trade and investment from the end of the Second World War, the expansion of world markets and the rise of transnational actors required far greater scrutiny. This led them to develop the concept of 'complex interdependence', drawing attention to the growing disjuncture between the authority of states and their capacity to exert such authority, in a world of increasingly powerful transnational actors and forces (Keohane and Nye 1977). Along the same lines, although from a critical theory perspective, Robert Cox wrote that the rise of a 'global class structure' has resulted from the internationalization of production by multinational, and increasingly transnational, corporations, leading to new patterns of social relations (Cox 1987). By the late 1980s, this restructuring of the IPE began to be strongly influenced by the concept of globalization. Stephen Gill and David Law, for example, sought to theorize and explain this emerging world order which they termed the *global* political economy:

> In a world where nuclear weapons, integrated capital markets, and global ecological threats have scant regard for national boundaries, a global concept is more and more needed to make sense of world society, and purposefully to act to shape it. (Gill and Law: 1988: xxiii)

Ngaire Woods (2001) and others (Jones 1995; Cerny 1996) asked whether globalization is diminishing the role of states in the world economy, and what role international institutions would be expected to play in managing globalization. While globalization is recognized as multifaceted in its drivers, processes and consequences, the changing nature of the IPE is regarded as one of its core features.

Applying a social constructivist approach, this chapter argues that certain narratives have been used to shape the IPE of global health in terms of influencing what is seen as the appropriate relationship between states and markets, the nature of the priority problems facing global health and their potential solutions, and the criteria used to allocate available resources. The remainder of this chapter explores these narratives in relation to the health care industry within the IPE; the commodification of the global health knowledge structure; and the impact of the IPE on health equity.

The Health Care Industry within the IPE

Health care is the prevention, treatment and management of illness, and the preservation of mental and physical well-being through the services offered by the medical and allied health professions. The UN International Standard Industrial Classification categorizes health care as consisting of hospital activities, medical and dental practice activities (e.g., physicians, nurses, midwives, pharmacists and physiotherapists), and 'other human health activities' such as services provided by scientific or diagnostic laboratories, pathology clinics, residential health facilities and other allied health professions, e.g. optometry, occupational therapy, speech therapy, chiropractics. Health care also includes the production of many categories of medical equipment, instruments and services, as well as biotechnology, diagnostic laboratories and substances, and drug manufacturing and delivery. Moreover, health care encompasses the financing of health care goods and services in the form of insurance providers and administrators.

The production structure of health care concerns what health care goods and services are produced, how they are produced, under what conditions, the terms by which they are sold and to whom. Health care expenditure worldwide totalled around US$5.5 trillion in 2010.[1] This figure represents over 10 per cent of gross domestic product (GDP) in most high-income countries. The sector is predicted to growth rapidly for two main reasons. First, a growing and ageing world population (figure 4.1) will mean increased demand. This not only includes high-income countries, but populations in emerging economies with unmet health care needs. Demand from emerging economies, notably Brazil, China and India, is expected to grow rapidly given a large and expanding patient pool, growing investment in health care infrastructure, rising household incomes and greater health awareness (Deloitte 2011).

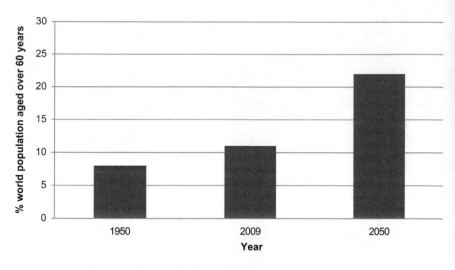

Source: United Nations (2009).

Figure 4.1 *Proportion of world population aged 60 years or over, 1950–2050*

For example, China is predicted to become the second largest health care market by 2014 (Ando 2011). Second, the development of new procedures and technologies will generate new patterns of demand. It is estimated that up to 8,000 new health technologies (mainly medical devices) come onto the US market alone annually (OECD 2005).

While total health care expenditure overall has been substantial and growing worldwide, what health care goods and services have been produced, by whom and for whom, have been strongly shaped by the IPE. The period from the Second World War to the 1970s was a period of marked expansion of health care systems in industrialized countries, funded either by state-funded health insurance or private insurance coverage through employment benefits (Quam 1989). Crises in the world economy from the early 1970s, punctuated by two oil crises and 'stagflation' (lower growth and employment coupled with high infla-tion), kindled widespread policy debate about the appropriate roles of the state and market in public services including health care. Given the rapid growth of health care costs, becoming the largest share of public expenditure in many countries, governments sought reforms aimed at controlling costs (Docteur and Oxley 2003). It was during this period that a broad set of policies, known as new public management (NPM), began to be influential. Under the banner of improving the delivery of public services, NPM proponents framed policy debates in economic terms, arguing above all for greater efficiencies through an increased role of the market and reduced state involvement, in the delivery of public services. NPM was closely akin to the then dominant economic theories of neo-liberalism which advocated, among other things, a 'minimalist' welfare state (Lynn 1998).

The ascendance of NPM-based ideas, in turn, profoundly influenced how health care goods and services have been produced and consumed worldwide. From the early 1980s, health systems in many OECD countries underwent a broad trend of reforms to contain costs by limiting the role of the state and encouraging its more efficient operation through market mechanisms. Policy debates focused, not on expanding access to health care, but on finding an affordable balance between the state and market in an era of financial austerity. In a broad range of high-income countries, including New Zealand, Sweden, the Czech Republic, the UK and the US, competition among health care providers was introduced (Docteur and Oxley 2003: 36–7). Policy innovations such as fundholding, contracting out, league tables and other performance indicators were developed to encourage the state to act more like a market. Efforts to relieve pressures on the public financing of health care also led to the introduction of user fees, private health insurance schemes and other cost-recovery methods (Ham 1997). As costs continued to rise, private health insurance schemes have also sought to achieve economies, according to Porter (2009: 109), by 'selecting healthier subscribers, denying services, negotiating deeper discounts, and shifting more costs to subscribers'. Overall, the IPE of health care reform since the 1980s has been dominated by an economic narrative, with its emphasis on cost containment and savings, rather than a concern for fair and equitable access to basic health care.

In low- and middle-income countries (LMICs), health reforms have played out in a similar fashion, although with harsher social consequences given more severe resource constraints, weaker capacity and, in many cases, greater health needs. The promotion of NPM-inspired policy ideas was led by external donors, notably the World Bank and IMF, initially in the form of structural adjustment programmes (SAPs) (Manning 2001). Similar to the narrative in high-income countries, the problem was defined as an oversized and inefficient state sector which, under the policy conditionalities required to receive financial assistance, governments had to commit to reforming through a package of policy measures. This package of policy measures gained support from a broad range of largely Washington-based institutions including USAID, the US Treasury Department and the World Bank. This so-called Washington Consensus had profound impacts on what health care goods and services were produced, how they were produced, and the terms by which they were accessed by patients. Regarding what health care goods and services were produced, World Bank-led SAPs focused on the belief that the state needed to be limited to financing and delivering an 'essential package' of health care services. This essential package was set out in two seminal reports, 'Health Care Financing in Developing Countries' (Akin et al. 1987) and the *World Development Report: Investing in Health 1993* (World Bank 1993). Coinciding with a substantial increase in World Bank lending for health development from the 1980s (Buse 1994), the *World Development Report 1993* (hereafter *WDR 1993*) set out what became a highly influential approach to financing and delivering public health and clinical services based on the concept of disability adjusted life years (DALYs). Arguing that, in many developing countries, '[p]ublic money is spent on health interventions of low cost-effectiveness . . . at the same time that critical and highly cost-effective interventions . . . remain underfunded' (World Bank 1993), the authors argued that more rational allocation of health resources could be achieved by measuring 'the cost-effectiveness of different health interventions and medical procedures – that is, the ratio of costs to health benefits (DALYs gained)' (World Bank 1993). A whole industry of health economists consequently sprang up, tasked with estimating the cost-effectiveness of varied health interventions, and health systems were reformed accordingly with a focus on delivering such essential packages:

> Ensuring basic public health services and essential clinical care while the rest of the health system becomes self-financed will require substantial health system reforms and reallocations of public spending. Only by reducing or eliminating spending on discretionary clinical services can governments concentrate on ensuring cost-effective clinical care for the poor. (World Bank 1993)

Within this framing of health sector reform in terms of the economic benefit that improved health could deliver, the *WDR 1993* gave particular attention to the roles of government and the market in health. It argued that there were three rationales for a government role in health: (a) when the poor cannot afford health care that would improve their productivity and well-being; (b) when promoting health is a pure public good or creates large positive externalities, and private markets would thus not produce them sufficiently; and (c) when market failure in health care and health insurance mean that government intervention can raise welfare by improving how those markets function (World Bank 1993: 52–3). Crucially however, through its advocacy of user fees, cost recovery, private health insurance, and public-private partnerships, the report called for limiting the role of the state to core public health and clinical services, and an enlarged role for the market and market forces. As well as calling for the domestic health reforms to prioritize certain interventions as part of an essential package, such as immunization, family planning, nutrition, tobacco and alcohol control, and HIV/AIDS and sexually transmitted disease treatment and prevention, the WDR 1993 called for health sector aid to be increased and focused on this strategy.

The production of health care goods and services in much of the developing world was consequently shaped by this economic narrative. While structural adjustment programmes, the WDR 1993 and other NPM-inspired policies sought to tackle the longstanding problem of inadequate and poor-quality health care, especially for the poor, in many parts of the world, evidence suggests that these measures led to 'an unprecedented decline of the health status of the poor' and much worsened health inequalities (Kanji et al. 1991; Loewenson 1996). In Tanzania, for example, the adoption of a series of 'adjustment measures' from 1981 onwards, including the reduction of government expenditure by introducing cost sharing in the health sector, has been accompanied by increased maternal mortality, chronic malnutrition and an erosion of capacity to implement HIV/AIDS intervention strategies (Lugalla 1995). The reduction in the share of public health and clinical services funded by government in seven Indian states, 'in accordance with the recommendations of the World Bank to confine the public sector's role to preventive care while the bulk of the curative services could be provided by the private sector', impacted severely on the poor who depended most heavily on publicly funded services (Prabhu 1994). Overall, by the mid-1990s, there was substantial criticism of the bluntness of SAPs and the so-called Washington Consensus (Sen and Koivusalo 1998). Evidence suggested that an oversized (and assumed inefficient) public sector was not the core problem in many LMICs but rather weak capacity (Batley and Larbi 2004) and a chronic lack of resources. Loewenson (1993) describes the introduction of World Bank/ IMF SAPs in more than forty African countries, with evidence indicating that the policies have been associated with increased food insecurity and under nutrition, rising ill-health, and decreased access to health care in two-thirds or more of the population of African countries that already lives below poverty levels. Similar findings were reported in Latin America and the Caribbean, where adjustments in macroeconomic policies had a negative effect on health indicators which lasted throughout the following decade (Franco-Geraldo et al. 2006). The introduction of cost-sharing measures, notably user fees, led particularly to a decline in access to health services. In Kenya, the introduction of fees resulted in a decrease of outpatient attendance by 27 per cent at provincial hospitals, 46 per cent at district hospitals, and 33 per cent at health centres (Willis and Leighton 1995). In Zambia and Ghana, outpatient attendance dropped by 35 per cent and 40 per cent respectively after fees were introduced (Biritwum 1994; Blas and Limbambala 2001).

This realization led to a renewal of the debate about the appropriate roles of the state and market, with the language shifting from achieving a 'minimalist' to an 'effective' state. The latter was defined as the capacity of state institutions

> to manage the business of the executive, judiciary and the legislature towards human development ends. Indicators of effective state capacity can be found in how national policies are made, services are delivered, markets are developed, justice and security provided, and rights are protected. Where this is done well – where large numbers of people benefit over time from development, when an economy grows and society is engaged in democratic processes and feels secure – then state capacity can be viewed as effective. (Gercheva et al. no date)

Within the health sector, criticism of the impacts of neo-liberalism shifted attention by the late 1990s to achieving an appropriate 'public-private mix' (Maynard 2005), with the narrative of limiting the state to essential functions unchanged. NPM ideas remained influential, with patients worldwide cast as a 'consumer' of health services who would best be served through increased competition among providers, contracting out of non-core services (e.g., catering, cleaning, laboratory services), managed care, new incentive mechanisms (e.g., bonuses for achieving targets) and performance indicators (Stocker et al. 1999). The creation of global public-private partnerships can be seen as an extension of this narrative, based on the claim that combining public service with competitive market forces would better achieve global health goals. In practice, however, the increased capacity of powerful economic interests to wield influence over international health policy resources raised further concerns (Bull and McNeill 2007).

Overall, health care reform over the past forty years has been profoundly shaped by a narrative that has sought to define the relative roles of the state and market using economic criteria. The IPE of health reform has been strongly influenced by neo-liberal-based ideas which, starting at the national level, have supported a shift towards 'the use of market mechanisms to finance and provide health services' (Kumaranayake and Lake 2002). In this way, the health sector reform agenda was constructed as fundamentally a problem of irrational resource allocation, economic inefficiencies and waste by oversized governments. However, this 'marketization' of health sector reform was underpinned by particular normative assumptions and values regarding the goals to be achieved (i.e. economic efficiency versus social justice) and the policy tools to achieve them (e.g., DALYs, cost-effectiveness measures). Moreover, while initially played out in individual countries, each with different health needs and resources, it is important to recognize the global nature of these policy reforms. While many policies originated in health reforms adopted at the domestic level, led by western industrialized countries, their core values and ideas permeated key donor agencies which, in turn, applied them across the developing world with profound consequences.

Global Restructuring in the Production of Health Goods

Health care goods comprise medical equipment, instruments and services, as well as biotechnology, diagnostic laboratories and substances, and drug manufacturing and delivery. The medical equipment and supplies industry alone, for example, is substantial, with total revenues worldwide of US$280 billion in 2009 (growing more than 8 per cent annually), and predicted to reach US$490 billion by 2016. Since the 1980s, there has been a global restructuring in the production of many health care goods, in part as a result of broader changes in the IPE, as well as the increased role of the market within the health sector. As Kumaranayake and Lake point out, '[m]arketization and increasing globalization in individual sub-markets within the health sector are beginning to generate a range of global markets for health-related goods and services' (Kumaranayake and Lake 2002: 80). This is well illustrated by the global restructuring of the pharmaceutical industry, with revenues of US$825 billion in 2010 (IMAP 2010), amid intense competition for new markets and greater economies of scale. New markets are led by the so-called 'pharmerging countries' (China, India, Brazil, Russia, Turkey, South Korea and Mexico), where demand is expected to grow 13–16 per cent per annum. Generating and competing for this new demand has led to increased concentration of ownership within the pharmaceutical and biotechnology industries since the 1990s, with thousands of mergers and acquisitions resulting in fewer and larger firms. In 1992 the top ten pharmaceutical companies (all with head offices in the US and Europe) accounted for roughly one-third of world revenue (Tarabusi and Vickery 1998; see also table 4.1). By 2002, this share had increased to one-half (Busfield 2005: 96) and by 2009 to around 55 per cent.[2] The industry has seen rapid growth during this

TABLE 4.1 World's ten largest pharmaceutical companies by sales (2010)

Rank	Company	Sales (US$ millions)	Headquarters
1	Pfizer	45,448	USA
2	Sanofi-Aventis	40,871	France
3	Novartis	38,455	Switzerland
4	GlaxoSmithKline	36,746	UK
5	AstraZeneca	31,905	UK
6	Merck & Co.	26,929	USA
7	Johnson & Johnson	22,520	USA
8	Eli Lilly & Co.	20,629	USA
9	Bristol-Myers Squibb	18,808	USA
10	Abbott Laboratories	16,486	USA

Source: Contract Pharma. Top 20 Pharmaceutical Companies Report. 2010. http://www.contractpharma.com/contents/view/33747.

period. In 2009, worldwide sales totalled US$808 billion (IMAP 2010), an increase from US$466 billion in 2003 (Busfield 2005: 96) and are projected to reach US$1.1 trillion by 2015 (IMS 2011).

Trends in mergers and acquisitions provide further evidence of increased concentration within the global pharmaceutical industry. In 2009–10, the pharmaceutical sector saw 1,021 deals valued at around US$210 billion. American and European companies secured the largest deals, while China saw the largest number of smaller deals. Of particular note have been companies seeking to expand into burgeoning emerging markets by acquiring domestic generic producers and manufacturing companies. These represented 50 per cent of the deals made during 2008–10 in emerging markets. Market analysts predict continued consolidation, further encouraged by low interest rates and availability of cash to spend (IMAP 2011).

Another feature of the IPE of the pharmaceutical industry is the growing importance of companies from emerging economies. While many US and European companies are actively targeting Brazil, Russia, India and China (BRIC) as the next big markets for their products, worth around US$132 billion in 2010 (Epsicom Healthcare Intelligence 2011), pharmaceutical companies within these countries are rapidly emerging as global players in their own right. The main focus of BRIC manufacturers is the production of cheaper versions of generic drugs, such as antiretrovirals and vaccines, notably for the developing world. For example, the BRIC countries already provide over 70 per cent of all vaccines purchased by procurement agencies. India is the world's third largest pharmaceutical producer (after the US and Japan) in terms of volume, and the 13th largest in terms of value (exports approximately US$10 billion in 2009–10). In 2011, the BRIC Ministers of Health issued a declaration pledging to help the poorest countries fight diseases through technology transfer and the supply of cheap and effective drugs (Azad 2011). In time, it is expected that the four countries will move from generics to the development of new drugs, posing further competition to established industry players. China, for example, moved the biotechnology, biomedicines, new vaccines, and advanced medical equipment sectors from the restricted to permitted categories for foreign investment, seen as a signal that they are 'strategic sectors and investments to be encouraged' (Shobert 2012). The production of certain biologicals (vaccines, cultures and other preparations made from living organisms and their products, intended for use in diagnosing, immunizing, or treating humans or animals, or in related research) has undergone similar restructuring. Of particular note is the blood products industry (see box 4.1), worth around US$13.4 billion in 2009, an increase of 16.7 per cent over 2007 (China Research and Intelligence 2011). The blood products

Box 4.1 The global restructuring of the blood products industry

Blood products contribute to saving millions of lives annually, improve life expectancy and the quality of life of patients suffering from life-threatening conditions, and support complex medical and surgical procedures. Global access to sufficient and safe blood products, however, is highly inequitable. More than seventy countries have a blood donation rate of less than 1 per cent of the population (estimated by WHO as the minimum needed to meet a country's basic requirements for blood). Ageing populations, more stringent donor selection criteria, inadequate storage and transportation, and poor blood stock management are cited by the WHO as contributing to the problem.

One of the worst treatment disasters in modern history took place in the 1980s with the widespread transmission through infected blood products of viral pathogens, in particular HIV and hepatitis B and C viruses. Blood-borne transmission of pathogens has highlighted the crucial importance of effective policies, quality systems, and legislative and regulatory frameworks in the collection, processing and supply of blood products, such as red cells, platelets and plasma for clinical use, and in the preparation of plasma for fractionation, as a raw material for the manufacturing of plasma-derived medicinal products, such as clotting factor concentrates and immunoglobulins, which are on the WHO Model List of Essential Medicines.

Recognizing the high risk of transmission of pathogens through transfusion of contaminated blood products, the World Health Assembly, in resolution WHA58.13, urged Member States to promote the development of national blood services based on voluntary non-remunerated donation and to enact effective legislation governing their operation. Blood services throughout the world are facing the daunting challenge of making sufficient supplies of blood products available to meet the needs of patients, while also ensuring the quality and safety of those products in the face of known and emerging threats to public health. The health-related Millennium Development Goals of reducing child mortality, improving maternal health and combating HIV/AIDS, malaria and other diseases cannot be achieved unless significant attention is paid to the availability, safety and quality of blood products.

The blood banking and blood products market is predicted to increase to US$36 billion by 2015. Much of the growth in the blood banking and blood products market is anticipated from the United States and Europe, as stated in a recent report published by Global Industry Analysts, Inc. The two regions collectively account for two-thirds of the global market. The market in Asia-Pacific is projected to grow between 4 and 5 per cent over the period 2001–10. In terms of product segment, the blood components and plasma products market is the largest with an estimated share of 81 per cent in 2008. The segment is also projected to be the fastest growing with a compound annual growth rate (CAGR) of 4.9 per cent over 2001–10. Automated blood collection and processing systems and unravelling prion-screening abilities of new assays are set to revolutionize the blood safety setup, both by increasing the blood quality and the quantity of blood collected through painless and sophisticated instruments. Several modifications in the purchasing system in the European market have provided hospitals with more bargaining power. The whole blood and cellular components market in Europe is estimated to be worth US$7.5 billion in 2008.

Sources: WHO (2009); Global Industry Analysts, Inc. (2010).

industry has become increasingly dominated by a few large producers including CSL Behring, Talecris Biotherapeutics, Grifols, Baxter International and Octapharma. The widespread transmission through infected blood products of viral pathogens during the 1980s, in particular HIV and the hepatitis B and C viruses, has led to the adoption of stricter policies by regulatory and health agencies. However, this has served to create further barriers to entry and, in turn, greater industry concentration (Global Industry Analysts, Inc. 2010). Today, blood donations collected across many countries are processed by this small number of producers whose blood products are then sold for use largely in high-income countries. Weak capacity and resource constraints have meant that there has been a chronic shortage of supplies of safe blood and blood products in low- and middle-income countries.

While health care services are, for the most part, delivered domestically, trade in health services is a growing industry. In the US, a substantial degree of integration and concentration has already occurred in the largely private health care market, leading to the formation of larger scale providers (Summer 2011). These companies have expanded abroad, finding opportunities in the wake of the deregulation and privatization within the health sectors of other countries. In the UK, for example, Mohan anticipated in the early 1990s the potential for multinational corporations to expand into the acute hospital sector and ancillary services, as part of the 'internationalization and commercialization' of the health sector depending on state policies regarding the provision of health care (Mohan 1991). A scathing review of the progressive privatization of the National Health Service (NHS), including increased service provision by large multinational companies, is also described by Pollock as part of a worldwide trend to make health care 'a commodity to be bought, rather than a right' (Pollock 2004).

A related development in the global restructuring of health care services is the crossborder delivery of care. This can take many forms – the migration of health care workers, the delivery of health care at a distance using various technologies (i.e. telemedicine), or the increased movement of patients across borders (McLean 2009). The latter, increasingly referred to as medical tourism, was predicted to be worth US$100 billion in 2012 (KPMG 2011). This growth will be partly driven by the inability of patients to obtain timely care locally. Longer waiting lists for procedures, deemed a 'lower priority' (e.g., hip replacements) by state-funded health care providers, was an initial motivation for patients to seek alternatives. In other cases, access to certain services may be restricted or not covered by basic health insurance (e.g., fertility treatment, cosmetic procedures). As NPM-driven health reforms have narrowed the range of health care services offered by the state, medical tourism has grown:

> With globalization, increasing numbers of patients are leaving their home communities in search of orthopaedic surgery, ophthalmologic care, dental surgery, cardiac surgery and other medical interventions. Reductions in health benefits offered by states and employers will likely increase the number of individuals looking for affordable medical care in a global market of privatized, commercial health care delivery. (Turner 2007: 303).

For lower-cost countries, such as China, Thailand and India, foreign patients have become a lucrative source of income. Despite estimates such as the one above, there is limited data available on current trends in medical tourism, which is likely to remain a limited proportion of total health care. Nevertheless, its growth is a further reflection of the restructuring of health care production spurred by its marketization across the world.

The Global Health Knowledge Structure

The knowledge structure of the IPE determines what knowledge is discovered, how it is stored, and who communicates it, by what means, to whom and on what terms. As Strange writes,

> power and authority are conferred on those occupying key decision-making positions in the knowledge structure, – on those who are acknowledged by society to be possessed of the 'right', desirable knowledge and engaged in the acquisition of more or it, and on those entrusted with its storage, and on those controlling in any way the channels by which knowledge, or information, is communicated. (Strange 1998: 121)

In global health, expenditure on research has more than quadrupled since 1998 to US$160.3 billion in 2005. While this growth has been seen as much welcomed, concerns have arisen about the source of these resources, the type of knowledge produced, and the influence of this knowledge on how global health needs are defined and addressed. Frustrations with the poor alignment between health research and need (measured by morbidity and mortality) were brought to the fore in the mid-1990s by the Global Forum for Health Research (2004) which observed that only 10 per cent of health research spending worldwide was being used to study the health needs of 90 per cent of the world's population. Known as the 10/90 gap, it was argued that most health research was being produced and consumed by high-income countries who were preoccupied with the health needs of the relatively wealthy and healthy. Correspondingly, there was a stark neglect of often more prevalent and severe health conditions suffered in the poorest countries:

> health research applied to the needs of low- and middle-income countries remains grossly under resourced in many areas and the term '10/90 gap', while not representing a current quantitative measure, has become a symbol of the continuing mismatch between needs and investments. (Global Forum for Health Research 2004)

While this disparity between the allocation of health research resources and need can be explained, in part, by the concentration by high-income governments on the health needs of their domestic populations, which would be different from aggregated global health needs, a closer look at the IPE of health research suggests more complex dynamics at play. First, the private sector undertakes a significant proportion of health research worldwide led by the pharmaceutical and biotechnology industries. As profit-seeking companies, they have pursued health research with a market-driven focus on health goods and services which promise the greatest economic return. Measured against the capacity to recoup research and development (R&D) costs, and to maximize profits, rather than measures, for example, based on improving human well-being or addressing health and social inequities, most private investments in health research have correspondingly targeted the concerns of certain population groups who can afford to pay over others who cannot. In the pharmaceutical industry, this R&D cost-recovery and concomitant profit-seeking behaviour has created global health inequities including the neglect of diseases promising insufficient economic returns (because of a patient group that is relatively small or unable to pay for treatment), overproduction of products for the relatively wealthy (such as drugs to treat obesity and impotence), and the disproportionate use of R&D resources to produce so-called 'me too' drugs which largely duplicate the action of existing drugs rather than develop genuinely new compounds (Gagne 2011).

Second, there is substantial evidence that major industries have sought to influence global health policy in ways that favour their own self-interests. Analysis of the tobacco industry has provided key insights, in particular, into how transnational tobacco companies have undermined the scientific process through funding and disseminating research, recruiting scientists as industry consultants, and undermining of public health institutions and scientists (WHO 2000; Samet and Burke 2001; Muggli et al. 2008). Tobacco industry-funded research has, for example, attributed the incidence of lung cancer to alternative explanations (e.g., indoor air pollution, diet, genetics), and cast doubt on the statistical significance of evidence on the health effects of second-hand smoke. Lexchin et al. (2003) investigated whether funding of drug studies by the pharmaceutical industry is associated with outcomes that are favourable to the funder and whether the methods of trials funded by pharmaceutical companies differ from the methods in trials with other sources of support. They found that there was systematic bias which favours products which are made by the company funding the research. Explanations include the selection of an inappropriate comparator to the product being investigated and publication bias (Lexchin et al. 2003). Brownell and Warner (2009) question whether the framing of global health issues in ways that serve tobacco industry interests can also be observed in the food industry. This seems to be confirmed by a study by Lesser et al. of research by the food industry on nutrition. The authors found that, when studies linking beverages to health are funded entirely by industry, the conclusions are four to eight times more likely to support the sponsor's commercial interest than studies with no industry funding (Lesser et al. 2007).

Third, along with governments such as the US, which devotes the largest proportion of its investment in research in the life sciences (US Congressional Budget Office 2007: XII), and industry, charitable foundations have become among the biggest institutional players in global health since the late 1990s, led by the Gates Foundation. As the world's largest funder of global health research, the Foundation has acquired unprecedented influence over what kind of knowledge is produced and for what purpose. Critics argue that the Foundation's penchant for developing biomedical research to treat infectious diseases has concentrated the world's best brain power to specific health problems and solutions (McCoy et al. 2010). Other donors have been guilty of the same, attracted by the public relations value of developing a new vaccine, distributing drug treatments or the ultimate goal of eradicating an entire disease (Shiffman 2008). However, as Stephen Matlin argues, 'We need a new model for public health for the 21st century, which acknowledges disease prevention and health promotion rather than [reliance on] the biomedical model of a drug for everything, to enable people to be healthier for longer' (cited in White 2004: 1064). Of particular concern is the neglect by research funders of understanding the broader social determinants of health and how, for example, structural factors create the social and environmental conditions which shape patterns of health and disease.

Fourth, complex alliances have emerged in health research among industry, governments, universities and non-state actors (notably charitable foundations and nongovernmental organizations) (US Congressional Budget Office 2007) that blur the boundaries between state and market interests. For governments and non-state actors, engagement with the private sector has been sought to supplement the limited availability of public resources and to gain access to R&D and entrepreneurial expertise. In addition, as Stopford and Strange (1991: 19–20) describe, the intensification of crossborder competition for both firms and states has led to closer interdependence between the two spheres in the form of government–company alliances. Within global health research, this has led to the formation of dozens of national and global public-private partnerships for health (Buse and Harmer 2007), a large number of which are focused on the development or improved use of drugs and vaccines to treat specific diseases (Buse and Walt 2000).

Many public health advocates have called for public-private partnerships to be located within 'a set of global norms and principles', and that the '[p]articipation of international agencies . . . be set within a comprehensive policy and operational framework within the organizational mandate' (Nishtar 2004). Many such partnerships have contributed significantly to social goals such as increased access to ARVs by the world's poor (Ramiah and Reich 2005) and developing treatments for neglected diseases (Buckup 2008). For industry, however, partnerships with governments and non-state actors can also serve a strategic purpose. Questions about conflicts of interest, and the compatibility of private interests and public policy goals, have grown as the result of reports of inappropriate conduct, selective data analysis and reporting, misrepresentation of study results, and attempts at scientific manipulation that have occurred with some industry-sponsored studies (DeAngelis and Fontanarosa 2010). Debate has focused on clinical trials and the pharmaceutical industry (Lundh et al. 2010), in particular, but the inappropriate influence of health research worldwide by other industries, such as tobacco (Muggli et al. 2008), food (Rowe et al. 2009; Nestle 2003) and alcohol (Anon 2011) has been widely revealed in recent years. In this context, industry funding of health research of public institutions directly, or through public-private partnerships, have been used as a means of increasing perceived credibility (Leutwyler 2000). Moreover, there is evidence to suggest that the external pressures created by industry funding can taint the scientific process. For example, a 2005 survey published in *Nature* of 3,247 US researchers who were publicly funded by the National Institutes of Health found that 15.5 per cent admitted to altering design, methodology or results of their studies due to pressure from an external funding source (Martinson et al. 2005). A similar study published in the *New England Journal of Medicine* found a comparable proportion of the 107 medical research institutions questioned willing to allow pharmaceutical companies sponsoring research to alter manuscripts according to their interests before they were submitted for publication (Mello et al. 2005).

One reflection of the emergence of a complex IPE of global health research and knowledge is its commodification, as a private good through the globalization of intellectual property rights (IPRs). IPRs have long protected ownership rights to creative works through national copyright, patent and trademark laws. Under the agreement on Trade-Related Intellectual Property Rights (TRIPS), a minimum standard of rights was required to be adopted across World Trade Organization (WTO) member states. There has been much criticism of the impact of the TRIPS agreement on public health, notably the adverse effect of patent protections on the affordability of medicines (Médecins Sans Frontières 2003). Within the context of the marketization of global health, the agreement must also be recognized as one that is framed by market economics. As health care goods and services have been increasingly framed within NPM-inspired policies, IPRs are a further expansion of the assertion of private ownership over knowledge as private goods, valued for their capacity to earn their owners profits (May 2009).

This economic framing of health knowledge contrasts, for example, with approaches that value its application foremost to improve human welfare. From this perspective, knowledge is seen as a public good to be openly shared and used. Challenges to the privatization of health knowledge can be seen in the movement to expand open access publishing (Barbour et al. 2006). A similar ethos lies behind the HINARI (Health InterNetwork Access to Research Initiative) Programme, established by WHO and major publishers, to enhance access by low-income countries to major collections of biomedical and health literature. More than 7,500 information resources (in 30 different languages) are now available to health institutions in 105 countries, areas and territories benefiting many thousands of health workers and researchers, and in turn, contributing to improve world health (WHO 2012).

In summary, the IPE of global health research is characterized by a complex of interdependent public and private interests which shape the processes by which knowledge is produced, what knowledge is produced, what knowledge is deemed legitimate, and how that knowledge is then used. This knowledge structure underpins the framing of global health problems in largely market economic terms, resulting in the prioritization of the health needs of the relatively well-off within and between countries.

The Global Political Economy of Health Inequities

Global health is replete with inequalities. The WHO Commission on the Social Determinants of Health begins its sobering report with the finding that a 'girl born today can expect to live for more than 80 years if she is born in some countries – but less than 45 years if she is born in others' (WHO 2008b: i). In their comprehensive study of global rates of adult mortality, Rajaratnam et al. find that adult males in Swaziland have nine times the probability of premature death than Cyprus. The rates of mortality in southern Africa are higher than rates were in Sweden in 1751 (Rajaratnam et al. 2010). Moreover, health inequalities have been increasing within as well as between countries. The former includes both high-income countries, such as the US (US CDC 2011) and

UK (Department of Health 2008b), and low-income countries such as China (Fang et al. 2010) and South Africa (Stuckler et al. 2011b).

Global health inequalities can be explained by complex combinations of biological, behavioural and environmental factors. Certain individuals or ethnic groups, for example, have a genetic predisposition to specific diseases such as sickle cell anaemia among people who are or were originally from Africa, parts of India and the Mediterranean, or Tay-Sachs Disease among Ashkenazi Jews. A population group with a high prevalence of smoking and excess alcohol consumption would expect to have a higher incidence of lung cancer, coronary heart disease and liver cirrhosis. Respiratory conditions can rise and fall for populations depending on their proximity to air-polluting factories. Together, biological, behavioural and environmental factors interact to produce many differences in health status within and across populations.

A global political economy approach to health inequalities, however, would ask to what extent biological, behavioural and environmental factors are shaped by interactions between the political and economic spheres. For instance, it is known that smoking prevalence is higher among populations of lower socioeconomic status. Such populations are characterized by lower educational attainment, higher rates of unemployment and a greater susceptibility to the marketing efforts of tobacco companies. Focusing on smoking behaviours alone, without understanding the factors that contribute to low socioeconomic status, can lead to the adoption of health interventions that may not effectively change such behaviours. Similarly, the reasons why populations might be more highly exposed to environmental pollutants may be changes in the world economy (e.g., rise of special economic zones) that impact on employment patterns and worker migration.

By focusing on the broad determinants of health, the global political economy also offers insights into health *inequities*. Two individuals with equal life chances and circumstances may decide to behave differently in terms of their lifestyle choices or seeking out health care. A resultant difference in health status can be described as a health *inequality*. Where individuals experience inequalities in health status due to differences in life chances or circumstances, particularly where such differences are due to unfairness or injustice, the resultant difference in health status can be described as a health *inequity* (Ruger and Kim 2006).

These inequities can also occur at the collective level. Total health care expenditure across the world was US$4.5 trillion in 2011, of which US$4.2 was consumed in OECD countries (OECD 2011). Countries in the highest quintile (20 per cent) spend more than 16 times the amount spent by the lowest quintile. The highest 5 per cent of the countries spend 4,492 per cent of the lowest quintile (UC Atlas of Global Inequality no date b). This inequality in health expenditure may be due to the decision by governments to allocate differing levels of resources to health care as opposed to other public expenditure, or for certain health care goods and services over others. However, countries also vary in their capacity to spend on health due to differing levels of wealth which, in turn, can be attributable to structural factors in the global political economy. Writing for the People's Health Movement, Legge argues that

> [t]he structured unfairness of the New World Order is not an accident. It is a direct consequence of the economic policies of the last two decades which have restructured the world economy in ways that favour the interests of the rich capitalist metropolis. These policies have been packaged separately for the poor world and the rich world. In the poor world they are called 'structural adjustment' and in the rich world they are labelled more generally as 'neoliberalism'. (Legge 2005)

Within this broader context of global structural inequity,

> [l]ack of access to care is associated with family and national poverty, user pays health care systems without insurance and privatization. Barriers to healthier ways of living include poverty, powerlessness, alienation and violence. Hazardous living environments are associated with family, regional and national poverty, war, lagging infrastructure development and environmental degradation. (Legge 2005)

Moreover, it is not just a lack of material power that sustains global health inequities. As described in this chapter, the capacity to frame health sector reform and the production of health goods and services within certain narratives, has advantaged certain interests over others. Neo-liberal-based economism has, for example, championed limiting the 'essential package' of state-provided health care to a minimum, investing the vast majority of health research funding to selected conditions and the development of biomedical interventions, and patent protecting new drugs to enable recovery of private investment. For private sector interests, such as the biotechnology industry, the future is believed to look rosy:

> The future perspective of medical industry seems to be immensely bright and encouraging for this industry in terms of the expected surge in global demand and upsurge in investments. Several trends such as globalization, continuous investments in research and development, newer techniques of drug development and discovery, product proliferation, mergers and acquisitions are the key drivers of this industry.

Increasing corporatization of Private Healthcare in the backdrop of a growing and affluent middle class is an emerging trend that has been pushing the growth of this industry. Health Insurance and Medical Tourism are the other significant trends, which are governing the global healthcare and medical industry. Most of the nations are now emphasizing on the accreditation of medical professionals so as to ensure legitimacy of the services provided by them. Robust advancement in the field of information technology will allow critical medical data to be processed and transferred quickly over larger distances, thereby saving time of both the patients and physicians in the speeding delivery of treatment. (Ernst & Young 2010)

Changing global patterns of health and disease, in short, reflect a complex picture that can be understood more fully through a global political economy lens. Although the world spends ever more on health care goods and services, the distribution of their production and consumption and, ultimately, their contribution to human welfare, is decidedly inequitable. These inequities can be explained by structural factors that shape material power, but also by mutually reinforcing ideational factors that allow certain narratives to dominate over others.

Conclusion

The international political economy of health concerns how health care goods and services are produced and consumed globally. This chapter has argued that an NPM-inspired narrative has dominated health sector reform since the 1980s which has focused on economic measures and tools to define the problem facing health systems, and the policy measures used to address them. This has led to a strong marketization of health systems, defined by a minimalized role for the state, and the introduction of market actors and market-based incentives into the public sector. A key feature of this was the manner in which the health sector reform agenda was constructed as the need to create a more rational allocation of resources. The advocacy of economic rationalism and evidence-based clinical decision making implied that this reform agenda was value-neutral. What we suggest, however, is that this was underpinned by normative assumptions concerning the value of economic efficiency over social justice, and that this served the interests of some over others, principally the 'haves' over the 'have-nots'. This is seen perhaps most clearly by the manner in which health research spending is disproportionately focused on the needs of the world's wealthiest populations, and the relative neglect of conditions suffered by the world's poor. Moreover, there has been a globalization of NPM-based ideas, leading to their application in high, middle and low-income countries, but also their transfer from the national to the regional and global levels. This has led to the restructuring of the production of health goods and services, framing of health development in terms of its impacts on the world economy, and the commodification of health knowledge as a private good. The narrative is sufficiently dominant that major players among bilateral donor agencies, UN organizations, multilateral financial institutions, charitable foundations and the scholarly community have all adopted such ideas and integrated them into their funding decisions and policy conditionalities in such a way that they often appear unchallenged and presented as 'common sense', rather than as a constructed narrative with distinctive normative underpinnings.

Most importantly, the ideas, interests and institutions that comprise 'global health' can be seen as extensions of what might be termed the 'global' political economy. Population health is seen, in this context, not as a value in itself, but as an input into the development of strong national economies and, by extension, the world economy. This starting point has led to a strong focus on health issues that pose the greatest threat to the world economy, namely potentially epidemic acute and severe infectious disease outbreaks. This chapter also suggests that significant health inequities are a reflection of such inequities in the global political economy.

CHAPTER FIVE

Global Health Governance

For over a decade a broad consensus has been emerging in both the academic and policy fields over the need for global health governance (GHG). Governance here is not the same as government, that is, a single law-making body that can impose its will on others. Rather it is a series of rules, norms and principles, some formal others less so, which are generally accepted by the key actors involved. Underpinning this consensus over the need for GHG is the globalization narrative: that the varied impacts of global change on human health have led to the need for more effective collective action. This has been particularly important as the capacity of national health systems, to protect and promote their domestic populations, have become more circumscribed. As many health determinants and outcomes have become transnational in nature, they have been beyond the control of national authorities alone to manage them. The protection and promotion of human health in an increasingly globalized world, in short, has prompted a search for better global health governance and a concern over the perceived shortcomings of the current governance framework.

Since the late 1990s, GHG has grown into a multidisciplinary subject of enquiry, initially emerging from within the public health field, but then attracting the attention of International Relations scholars. The term has been applied somewhat broadly and, at times, without clear definition. In large part, this has been because the study of GHG is closely intertwined with its practice. Emerging separately from the study by International Relations scholars of global governance more generally, this has resulted in weak theorizing and an entangling of description with prescription. The study of GHG, as a result, has been strongly problem-based, normatively-driven and highly contested. This chapter examines how normative frameworks have defined the conceptualization and practice of GHG to date. It is argued that different frameworks have been influential over time, varying across global health issues and interests. The ascendance of, and contestation among, these frameworks have, in turn, shaped how problems in GHG have been defined, what goals GHG is intended to pursue, and what means are deemed appropriate to pursue those goals. Moreover, it is argued that certain dominant normative frames are themselves factors that have led to the problems currently faced in GHG. In this sense, normative frameworks have defined both the analytical boundaries of GHG as a scholarly field, and its practical application in protecting and promoting population health in a globalizing world. The argument in this chapter is that the lack of progress in GHG is not simply an administrative, scientific or technical shortfall, but are a result of it being a highly contested realm of ideas, interests and institutions.

From International to Global Health Governance

Health has played a key part in the history of the human species. Patterns of health and disease across the centuries have played an integral role in the formation and interaction of societies, the rise and fall of civilizations, the migration of populations across the globe, the development of new knowledge and technologies, and the accumulation of wealth and political power. As Paul Basch describes, '[s]ince the earliest days, articles of booty or commerce, along with genes, infectious agents, and ideas, have been distributed within and between human populations' (Basch 1999: 6). In this sense, health has been 'global' from the formation of human social groups and their migration across geographical territories. In a stricter sense, however, the distinction between *international* and *global* health can be understood in terms of the degree to which health determinants and outcomes are limited by political geography and, in particular, the territorial boundaries of the states' system. The Peace of Westphalia in 1648, which ended the Thirty Years War and created the European states system, formed the basis of contemporary international relations. The state, as it exists today, was established as a compulsory political institution that maintains a monopoly over the legitimate use of force within a certain territory. The principle of state sovereignty has meant that anarchy, or the absence of a higher authority, has governed the states' system. Health governance, in this context, has been formed primarily at the state level, with national governments holding recognized authority to set and uphold rules and policies to achieve agreed health goals. International health governance, in this sense, concerned how nationally-based health authorities cooperated across their territorial jurisdictions to pursue shared goals through the establishment of rules and policies, as well as corresponding institutions. The focus of international health governance has remained the state, its authority over a given geographical territory, and its responsibility to protect and promote the health of the population within that territory.

In practice, international health governance has been defined by how major states have perceived the need to pursue shared health goals. During the nineteenth century, cooperation focused on facilitating trade interests by minimizing the interference caused by selected epidemic diseases and efforts to control them. The international surveillance, monitoring and reporting of such diseases remained the focus of health cooperation following the First World War and up to the end of the Second World War. Amid major disease outbreaks after 1945, and the movement to create national health services in Europe and elsewhere, advocates of liberal institutionalism argued that health should form a pillar of postwar functionalism. Yet, even then, the creation of the World Health Organization (WHO) was something of an afterthought, omitted from the United Nations Conference on International Organization of 1945. The WHO was finally established in 1948 and, over the next several decades, the scope of international health activities broadened in correspondence with the objective of 'the attainment by all people of the highest possible level of health' (WHO 1946). The greatest achievement of international health governance to date can be seen as the eradication of smallpox in 1979.

While international health activities increased in scope and scale, the degree to which there was increased governance is unclear. Indeed, public health narratives focused on national health strategies rather than international cooperation. Legal instruments governing international health activities remained few and far between led by the International Health Regulations. More numerous were 'soft law' instruments such as the International Code on the Marketing of Breastmilk Substitutes, Essential Drugs List and Declaration of Alma Alta on Primary Health Care. Additional intergovernmental organizations were established with international health activities such as UNICEF, UNFPA and UNDP, while the World Bank began to lend for health development in the 1990s. As described below, more players did not necessarily mean more governance. Indeed, over time, international health seemed to be characterized by less rather than more governance as individual institutions pursued their own agendas in a highly uncoordinated fashion in the absence of a higher authority or agreed goals.

In this context, the rise of GHG, as a concept and practice, can hardly be described as a progression from international health governance. If the latter existed to a limited extent, it is arguable that GHG exists at all. In part, this is a problem of definition. As described in chapter 1, the term global health has become all-encompassing and, as a result, poorly defined. GHG has correspondingly suffered from imprecision in terms of what it should look like and the domains in which it should operate. At the same time, GHG is much sought after as part of a narrative which emphasizes a holistic view of health as affected by, and affecting, the world as a whole. This narrative encompasses the rising importance of forces that circumvent, or even ignore, the territorial boundaries of states and which include many health determinants and outcomes (Brown et al. 2006). As such movements have intensified and extensified (increased geographical reach) (Held et al. 1999), the limitations of international health governance have become stark. In some cases, strengthening of international health governance is needed. In other cases, the world's health needs to be understood and governed in its entirety from a global perspective.

The rapid proliferation of literature on GHG since the 1990s reflects a broad consensus that there is a need to strengthen collective action to address global health concerns. While angst about the shortcomings of GHG has been largely prompted by what John Kirton calls 'real world concerns' (Kirton 2009), the specific problems identified and given priority in contemporary debates, and the universe of solutions deemed available to address them, have been strongly shaped by particular normative frameworks. The remainder of this chapter examines the social construction of GHG. This reveals that there are competing frameworks which have led to an often confused, and invariably contested, agenda for reform. The proliferation of global health initiatives since the late 1990s can be explained, above all, by this contestation. More critical reflection of how such frameworks are shaping the study and practice of GHG is urgently needed.

Security from Contagion: GHG to Prevent, Control and Treat Acute and Severe Epidemic Diseases

The early history of health cooperation has been defined foremost by a focus on infectious diseases framed in terms of fighting contagion from acute and severe epidemic diseases originating abroad (Moore 2008). This is perhaps understandable given that diseases which spread across national borders, especially those causing relatively high rates of morbidity and mortality (severe), in a relatively short period of time (acute), epitomized the need for effective collective action by states. The fourteen International Sanitary Conferences held from 1851 were largely convened for this purpose. Prompted by deadly cholera epidemics raging across Asia and Europe during the nineteenth century, European governments sought to standardize measures and develop at-the-border responses. The resultant International Sanitary Conventions were telling, not only in the selected diseases covered (namely cholera, plague, yellow fever), but the circumscribed range of functions mandated – the monitoring and surveillance of these diseases, collecting and sharing of data, and 'at-the-border' measures to prevent their spread (e.g., quarantine). For European governments, contagion was deemed to originate from 'out there' and could be stopped at the border with standardized international quarantine regulations. At the same time, the governance created was minimalist, designed to limit interference with the burgeoning political and economic ties between European countries and their colonized territories. The conventions, for example, did not agree collective action to aid endemic countries to prevent the occurrence and spread of outbreaks. Nor did the conventions deal with other disease areas or health conditions. This minimalist form of governance, focused on acute and severe epidemic diseases, and framed in terms of the spread of contagion from 'out there' to 'over here', extended to the functions of the International Office of Public Health created in 1909 and the League of Nations Health Organization formed in 1923, focused on epidemic control, quarantine measures and drug standardization.

The renewed attention to emerging and re-emerging diseases in the late twentieth century mirrors this earlier history. Contemporary globalization has been characterized by intensified crossborder flows of people and other life forms, goods and services, and knowledge and ideas. These flows, in many cases, have led to profound global environmental change. As history has shown, social change and commensurate shifts in the behaviour of human populations have led to changing patterns of health and disease. Amid the diverse and wide-ranging changes to human health, however, the narrative has privileged acute and severe infectious disease outbreaks with epidemic potential, while other health conditions remain relatively unremarked upon. Moreover, the framing of such diseases as contagion from abroad, to be contained using 'at the border' measures, has regained popularity. In the US, Markel and Stern describe the 1993 adoption by President Bill Clinton of the National Institutes of Health Revitalization Act, which amended the Immigration and Nationality Act of 1988, adding HIV infection as a criterion to keep out immigrants. The policy was one in a long history of efforts to 'shield the US against external pathogens' (Markel and Stern 2002: 757). The US government has been far from alone in seeking to exclude migrants on the basis of disease risk. According to the European AIDS Treatment Group, seventy-four countries have some form of HIV-specific travel restrictions, twelve of which ban HIV positive people from entering for any reason or length of time. The most common reasons used are to protect public health and avoid possible costs associated with care, support and treatment of people living with HIV (UNAIDS 2008). In relation to other diseases, in the UK, the then opposition Conservative Party published *Before It's Too Late: A new agenda for public health* in 2003, which called for the pre-screening of people seeking permission to remain in the country, and the detention of asylum seekers, to ensure they posed no risk of transmitting an infectious disease to the public; would not create undue demand on finite health resources, and did not create a long-term drain on the public purse (cited in Coker 2003). What Priscilla Wald calls the 'outbreak narrative', following the emergence of HIV/AIDS in scientific publications and the mainstream media (Wald 2007) has also shaped health governance at the global level. As described in chapter 6, security concerns have been influential in framing global health since the early 1990s. The end of the Cold War, and the acceleration of globalization, served to cast a spotlight on health issues deemed to pose 'new security' concerns. Acute and severe epidemic diseases, sometimes combined with rising concerns over bio-terrorism, served to define debates about the shortcomings of GHG in particular ways.

The revision of the International Health Regulations (IHRs) is a good illustration of this. The narrowing scope of the IHRs, with the diseases covered reduced from six to three (cholera, plague and yellow fever) by 1983 following the eradication of smallpox, sat in direct contrast with the increased risk from a growing number of diseases in an era of globalization. While the World Health Assembly (WHA) instructed the WHO Secretariat to begin a process of revision in 1995, proceedings stumbled along anaemically over the ensuing decade. One stumbling block was whether to include the threat of bio-terrorism. Even prior to the anthrax attacks of 2001, the US government was allocating funding to improving bio-terrorism preparedness and response capabilities at the federal and state levels (Fidler 2004). The creation of the Office of Health Affairs (including its Health Threats Resilience Division) within the US Department of Homeland Security, was part of these efforts: 'The Office of Health Affairs (OHA) is at the intersection of homeland security and public health, better known as health security. All threats to the homeland have health consequences' (Parker 2011).

The US government's desire to include acts of bio-terrorism within the revised IHR, as an extension of the so-called War on Terror, was opposed by other governments who saw it as a technical framework for addressing disease outbreaks. As one negotiator from Asia stated,

One of the main issues for us throughout the formal negotiations was the definition of 'disease' in the IHR. North America and Europe really wanted to include terrorism and terrorist events but our government objected to this notion. There was no need to include this. (Kamradt-Scott in press)

The shift from political indifference, to what Fidler calls a 'governance tipping point for global infectious disease control', was prompted by the SARS (severe acute respiratory syndrome) outbreak of 2002–3 (Fidler 2004). This led to substantial progress by the Intergovernmental Working Group (IGWG) in 2004 and 2005, with the revised text adopted by the WHA in May 2005. Under the terms of the IHRs (2005), governments have until July 2012 to develop and maintain 'core capacities' to detect, assess, notify and respond to 'public health emergencies of international concern' (PHEIC). Fidler argues that this represents 'a new way of working', marking a paradigmatic shift from state-based Westphalian to post-Westphalian GHG.

As well as the revision of the IHRs, the security framing of GHG is reflected in the creation of the Global Health Security Initiative (GHSI) in 2001 (box 5.1). Following the attack on the World Trade Center on 11 September 2001, former US Secretary of Health and Human Services Tommy Thompson suggested that countries fighting terrorism should meet to share information and coordinate their efforts to improve global health security. The resultant initiative is 'an informal, international partnership among like-minded countries [Canada, the US, UK, European Union, France, Germany, Italy, Japan and Mexico] to strengthen health preparedness and response globally to threats of chemical, biological, radio-nuclear terrorism (CBRN) and pandemic influenza' (GHSI no date). Since 2001, ministers have broadened the scope of the GHSI mandate to include the public health threat posed by pandemic influenza.

Securitization of GHG also framed the renewal of public health systems worldwide as they moved to countering health threats. In the UK, the Health Protection Agency (HPA) was formed in 2003 as an independent agency with the mandate to protect the public from threats to their health from infectious diseases and environmental hazards. The agency combines public health and scientific knowledge, research and emergency planning within one organization – and works at international, national, regional and local levels. It also supports and advises other organizations that play a part in protecting health. It identifies and responds to health hazards and emergencies caused by infectious disease, hazardous chemicals, poisons or radiation. It gives advice to the public on how to stay healthy and avoid health hazards, provides data

Box 5.1 Global Health Security Initiative

On November 7, 2001, the Canadian Minister of Health hosted the first Ministerial Meeting to discuss global health security. Ministers called for concerted global action to strengthen public health preparedness and response to the threat of international biological, chemical and radio-nuclear terrorism. They agreed to forge a partnership to address issues of protecting public health and security globally, and to work together in the following areas:

- To explore joint cooperation in procuring vaccines and antibiotics.
- To engage in a constructive dialogue regarding the development of rapid testing, research in variations of vaccines, and our respective regulatory frameworks for the development of vaccines, and in particular smallpox vaccines.
- To further support the World Health Organization's disease surveillance network and WHO's efforts to develop a coordinated strategy for disease outbreak containment.
- To share emergency preparedness and response plans, including contact lists, and consider joint training and planning.
- To agree on a process for international collaboration on risk assessment and management and a common language for risk communication.
- To improve linkages among laboratories, including level four laboratories, in those countries which have them.
- To undertake close cooperation on preparedness and response to radio-nuclear and chemical events.
- To share surveillance data from national public health laboratories and information on real or threatened contamination of food and water supplies along with information on risk mitigation strategies to ensure safe food supplies.

Source: GHSI[1]

and information to government to help inform its decision making, and advises people working in health care. It also makes sure the nation is ready for future threats to health that could happen naturally, accidentally or deliberately (i.e. bio-terrorism). The creation of the European Centre for Disease Prevention and Control (ECDC) in 2005 extended this model to the regional level. Based in Stockholm, the purpose of the EU agency is described as 'to identify, assess and communicate current and emerging threats to human health posed by infectious diseases' (ECDC 2004).

In summary, framing the challenge of GHG primarily as one of preventing and controlling the spread of acute and severe epidemic diseases across national borders is closely aligned with realist conceptions of international relations. It assumes that contagion can be contained 'at the border' with sufficient national capacity and, by extension, global institutional structures that support and reinforce those capacities. The establishment of security-defined health protection agencies at the national, regional and global levels, and the allocation of resources for governance functions focused on the surveillance, monitoring and reporting of disease outbreaks, is an expression of this framework. Authority resides firmly with the state, either with public health systems with the power to screen, isolate and, where necessary, exclude individuals and populations from crossing a national border; or with national security agencies tasked with planning for major health threats to ensure effective response, resilience and 'surge capacity'. This casting of global health in military terms has been most prominent in the US, where the threat from bio-terrorism has been a core component of governance arrangements. However, the 'outbreak narrative' has been readily apparent in a wide range of other countries, shaping how they define collective action problems in global health.

Western Biomedicine's Search for Magic Bullets: Fighting Diseases with Medical Science

Spectacular advances in medical science since the nineteenth century has bred an understandable belief that, with the right knowledge and its application, interventions can be developed that will transform health worldwide. These are not unfounded claims. Medical devices such as scanners, implants and dialysis machines, technologies such as x-ray, ultrasound and laser surgery, and drugs such as penicillin, insulin and vaccines have revolutionized health care and contributed significantly to improving population health. By extension, investing in more and more of the same it would seem would be a wise strategy to effectively address the biggest health problems facing the world. It is this belief in the promise of medical science that has inspired the work of many major global health institutions, led by the Bill and Melinda Gates Foundation (BMGF). In scoping out the foundation's work, Bill Gates reportedly consulted the World Bank book, *Disease Control Priorities in Developing Countries* (DCP1) (Jamison et al. 1993),[2] a companion document of the *World Development Report 1993* based on findings from the Disease Control Priorities Project (DCPP). As part of the Bank's emphasis on using economic rationales to inform priority setting in health development policy (see chapter 4), the book identified '25 priority conditions in low- and middle-income developing countries and assessed their public health significance and the cost-effectiveness of preventive and patient management interventions' (World Bank 2006). As described by the World Bank, '[t]he impact of the two publications was to stimulate national and international debate on health-sector investments, and to catalyze intensive work on the estimation of the disease burden and the cost-effectiveness of specific health interventions. Both publications have become reference works used extensively by policymakers, international development agencies, and academic institutions' (World Bank 2006). In 2006, a second edition (DCP2) was published that included updated information about the global burden of diseases brought about by tobacco, alcohol, psychiatric disorders, and injury and the cost-effectiveness of related interventions. This was accompanied by two influential volumes, *Priorities in Health* and *Global Burden of Disease and Risk Factors*, the latter providing 'a snapshot of health conditions of mankind at the dawn of the 21st century. GBD is a single source of up-to-date data on the global burden of disease, as well as the underlying methodologies for the cost-effectiveness calculations and conclusions presented in DCP2' (World Bank 2006).

Gates was reportedly inspired by these analyses. At the annual World Economic Forum in Davos, Switzerland in 2003, he announced the first round of the BMGF's Grand Challenges in Global Health. As Varmus et al. describe, 'The Global Health initiative was proposed by the . . . Gates Foundation . . . on the assumption that, with greater encouragement and funding, contemporary science and technology could remove some of the obstacles to more rapid progress against diseases that disproportionately affect the developing world (Varmus et al. 2003: 398). Since 2005, the Grand Challenges in Global Health initiative (see box 5.2) has provided US$458 million 'to overcome persistent bottlenecks in creating new tools that can radically improve health in the developing world.[3]

In fairness, the Gates approach follows a long line of technocratic initiatives in health cooperation. The decades-long debate, between pursuing biomedical fixes to the world's health problems (referred to as the search for magic bullets) and addressing the social determinants of health such as poverty and inequality (Lee 2004) remains ongoing. What is remarkable about the Gates Foundation, however, is the unprecedented scale (measured by volume of funding) of support for finding grand scientific solutions. By directing such huge resources into biomedical research, critics argue that distortions in GHG are being created (Beckett 2010). This is apparent, above all, in the predominance of initiatives focused on three diseases – HIV/AIDS, tuberculosis and malaria (Shiffman 2006). A slew of global public-private partnerships in health, formed from the late 1990s, are framed by the belief that substantial progress could be achieved by harnessing the innovation and resources of the private sector in the public interest (Buse and Walt 2000). These included, for example, the non-profit Medicines for Malaria Venture

Box 5.2 What is a Grand Challenge?

On 1 May 2003, in a solicitation widely advertised in the developed and developing world, a grand challenge was described as 'a call for a specific scientific or technological innovation that would remove a critical barrier to solving an important health problem in the developing world with a high likelihood of global impact and feasibility'. Throughout the process of developing the grand challenges, the board struggled with how best to define them. A grand challenge is envisioned as distinct from a simple statement of one of the many 'big problems' in global health, such as HIV/AIDS, malnutrition, the lack of access to medical care, or the lack of adequate resources. A grand challenge is meant to direct investigators to a specific scientific or technical breakthrough that would be expected to overcome one or more bottlenecks in an imagined path toward a solution to one or preferably several significant health problems. To satisfy this intent, a successful proposal would need to foresee a critical path of this type to get past a clearly defined roadblock. This formulation worked most effectively for those medical problems that are well enough understood to allow a description of what needs to be done, even if we do not yet know precisely how to do it. Thus, although the Grand Challenges initiative would ideally inspire unexpected and even radical solutions, the board also recognized the advantages of being able to envision solutions that have a high likelihood of being successful. The constraint of describing a 'critical path past a bottleneck' ruled out the broad field-building and exploratory research that usually underlies breakthroughs. Capacity building is another important approach (for example, increasing the number of biomedical research laboratories in the developing world, providing greater financial support for the study of global health or expanding professional training programs in global health) but beyond the purview of the program.

Source: Excerpt from Varmus et al. (2003: 398–9).

which 'manages the world's largest malaria research and development portfolio, covering the innovation spectrum from basic drug discovery to late-stage development' (Bathurst and Hentschel 2006). As Garrett writes, new funding has been 'directed mostly at specific high-profile diseases – rather than at public health in general' (Garrett 2007: 15).

Decisions about where not to allocate scarce funding resources also influence the nature of GHG. This has led to the neglect of some diseases over others depending on whether or not funders deem them amenable to biomedical scientific breakthroughs. The approach goes against conditions which require what are known as 'complex interventions' (health interventions involving multiple interacting components and non-linear causal pathways) (Petticrew 2011), some components perhaps lacking the glamour of medical science yet offering potentially greater health gains. Water and sanitation is a case in point. Toilets and sewers are hardly glamorous at the best of times, but when competing with vaccine development, for example, are often passed over by major funders despite the opportunity to reduce morbidity and mortality significantly from water-borne diseases. In 2011 the Gates Foundation recognized the need to champion more basic health needs with a US$10 million grant to develop 'innovative solutions' for sanitation in poor urban areas (Michler 2011).

The Search for Scientific Rationality: The Ascendance of the Evidence-based Approach in GHG

Closely aligned with the biomedical model in GHG has been the rise of evidence-based approaches, with certain types of 'evidence' and methodologies given privileged authority and legitimacy. The rise of evidence-based approaches in the early 1990s within high-income countries stemmed largely from a desire to agree and standardize 'best practice' in clinical medicine amid a dizzying array of knowledge and procedures. As well as improving patient care, identifying best practice would help optimize scarce resources. This desire to better inform medical practice has led to the elevation of the systematic review, in particular, as a methodology ostensibly aimed at reducing bias in clinical decision making (Petticrew 2001). Within biomedical research, evidence hierarchies have been developed to reflect the relative authority of a range of data sources, with randomized control trials (see figure 5.1) generally deemed the 'gold standard' of medical evidence, and expert opinion and anecdotal experience ranked lowest. While evidence-based medicine or practice has recognized that many aspects of health care depend on normative values (such as assessments of quality of life and value-of-life), its focus has been on aspects of medical practice that are subject to scientific methods that seek to quantitatively measure and predict the outcomes of different medical treatments (Greenhalgh 1997).

As Béhague et al. argue, the evidence-based medicine framework has since become institutionalized worldwide (Béhague et al. 2009). A whole industry has sprung up, not only to generate the prescribed evidence, but to systematically review such evidence. In 1993, the Cochrane Collaboration of more than 100 countries was formed to serve as a global repository of such reviews (around 4,600 to date). Based on 'the best available research evidence', the Cochrane Reviews are 'internationally recognized as the benchmark for high quality information about the effectiveness of health care'.[4] In low- and middle-income countries, where pressures on resources were even greater, the lack of

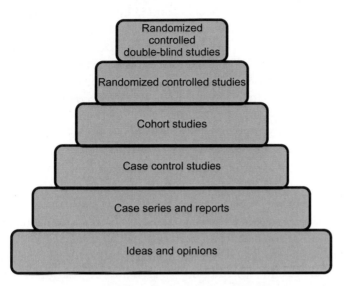

With kind permission from Springer Science+Business Media:
Oncology: an Evidence-based Approach, Chang et al. (eds.), 2005,
chapter one, page 5, figure 1.1, E. DeVoto and B.S. Kramer.

Figure 5.1 *Heirarchy of evidence in evidence-based medicine*

accurate, complete and comparable health information was recognized
as hindering health development. Addressing this gap was seen to be
especially important for addressing the often skewed allocation of
health resources within and across countries, and across different
disease areas.

Alongside the rise of evidence-based medicine have been efforts to
extend this approach to policy making known as evidence-based policy.
This development has been observable across many government sectors
and governments. The approach, once again, seeks to improve the
quality of decision practice by relying on the best evidence available, as
opposed to 'opinion-based policy, which relies heavily on either the
selective use of evidence (e.g., on single studies irrespective of quality)
or on the untested views of individuals or groups, often inspired by
ideological standpoints, prejudices, or speculative conjecture' (Davies
2004). By the mid-1990s, along with systematic reviews, the 'best' evidence in global health policy was deemed to be economic. This was
epitomized by the influence of the Global Burden of Disease Project,
hailed as 'a major landmark in public health and a foundation for
rational policy making and critical priority setting'[5] In 1998, project

co-lead Christopher Murray was appointed by incoming WHO Director-General Brundtland as Director of the Global Programme on Evidence for Health Policy. He later became Executive Director of the Evidence and Information for Policy (EIP) Cluster of the WHO in 2001 (Murray and Lopez 1996). During his tenure, major emphasis was placed on improving health metrics, defined as measures to better understand the current state of population health using rigorous, comparable, and current scientific measurement of trends in diseases, injuries, risk factors, and death, analysing data across countries and over time. These measures are then used by decision makers to understand what is making people sick and therefore to design appropriate prevention programmes and to best target the delivery of drugs, vaccines and other interventions. Since 2000, the emphasis on the generation and application of health metrics has continued to grow. After leaving the WHO in 2003 and a period back at Harvard University, Murray formed the Institute of Health Metrics and Evaluation at the University of Washington in 2008 with major funding from the Gates Foundation. The Institute is a major partner in the Health Metrics Network (HMN), established in 2005, to strengthen national health information systems.[6]

In a world of finite health resources and growing demand, achieving the most 'bang for your buck' is a stark reality. Improvements in data can better measure and compare health needs within and across different populations. Moreover, longitudinal data (that is, data collected over time) can be used to assess the relative effectiveness of specific treatments, interventions and policies. However, what has been apparent since the 1980s has been a narrowing of the type of data and methodologies used by policy makers. The elevation of biomedical, quantitative and economic 'evidence' has become the rationale for the creation of major institutions dedicated to generating and applying such data, while GHG initiatives have relied on their results to make fundamental decisions about the allocation of resources to specific population groups and for specific purposes. This is evident in the proliferation of initiatives intended to improve the evidentiary basis by which decision making can take place. The standing and influence of individuals and institutions with such expertise, in turn, have been elevated within GHG. Moreover, such evidence is seen to play a positive role in strengthening GHG itself. As Murray and Frenk write, 'In addition to its technical value, the explicit assessment of reform efforts [using GBD data] contributes to transparency and accountability' (Murray and Frenk 2010: 99).

Overall, the influence of the evidence-based approach has been profound in GHG (though on some of the limits of this approach, see

Kristiansen and Mooney 2004). Biomedical data, combined with economic analyses, have come to dominate policy making along with calls for better quality information on which to make decisions. With sufficient high-quality information, advocates of the evidence-based approach argue that decisions can then be made about health priorities and the allocation of resources without recourse to opinion and beliefs. Implicit in this is an attempt to de-politicize health. But such an approach cannot be divorced from normative concerns. The basis on which empirical research is conducted is underpinned by normative concerns over the subject of research, the question asked and appropriate methods, while 'evidence' can be used, mis-used and (re-)interpreted (not always consciously) to fit a variety of desired outcomes.

Tackling the Social Determinants of Health: Moving beyond Health Institutions

In contrast with a focus on the health sector and, more narrowly, selected disease areas, there have been calls to reform GHG to better tackle the social determinants of health. The greatest strides in improving population health during the nineteenth and twentieth centuries were the result of improved living and working conditions, namely improved access to clean water and sanitation, better housing and nutrition, and improved education and socioeconomic status (Cutler and Miller 2005; Marmot 2007). Access to health care has been important, of course, but relatively less so than better social conditions. These lessons, as argued by the Chairman of the WHO Commission on the Social Determinants of Health (CSDH) Michael Marmot, are apt for addressing contemporary health inequities:

> The poor health of the poor, the social gradient in health within countries, and the marked health inequities between countries are caused by the unequal distribution of power, income, goods, and services, globally and nationally, the consequent unfairness in the immediate, visible circumstances of peoples' lives – their access to health care, schools, and education, their conditions of work and leisure, their homes, communities, towns, or cities – and their chances of leading a flourishing life . . . Together, the structural determinants and conditions of daily life constitute the social determinants of health and are responsible for a major part of health inequities between and within countries. (WHO 2008b: 5)

With health inequities as the normative starting point, advocates of the social determinants of health approach have sought to reform existing GHG institutions to deal more effectively with broader factors beyond the health sector. As described above, GHG to date has been strongly shaped by the biomedical model with many organizations dedicated to addressing specific diseases, health system inputs or behaviours. In contrast, the CSDH argues for a more holistic approach for achieving 'good' GHG beginning with the reform of the multilateral system as a whole (see figure 5.2). Health policy is seen as requiring closer links with other policy realms, notably foreign and economic policy. For example, the health impact of trade agreements would need to be tackled as part of trade negotiations (Smith et al. 2009) and increased interagency collaboration with other UN bodies, such as the WTO and FAO, is advocated.

The importance of political voice is central to the social determinants of health approach. At the global level, the CSDH argues that the WHO should be the leading advocate for health within core global governance institutions (Bell et al. 2010). However, the question of who should be given a voice in global health policy, and how this should be institutionalized, has been the subject of growing debate. What forms of representation are needed to reflect the emerging global health polity? Major global health initiatives have adopted different governance structures (see table 5.1). Some argue that the WHO, by

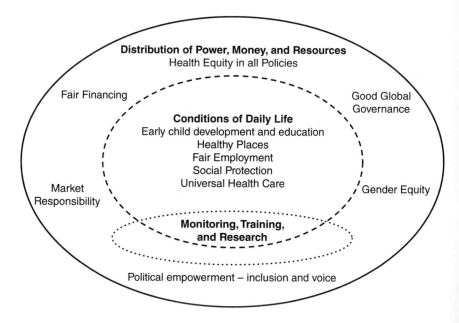

Source: Bell et al. (2010: 479). Reprinted with permission, John Wiley and Sons.

Figure 5.2 *Commission on Social Determinants of Health: Areas for action*

virtue of its 192 member states, is the most universally representative and should thus be given the lead role in global health policy. The erosion of its mandate and authority since the 1980s is seen as a reflection of the concentration of power in the hands of major donor governments at the expense of low- and middle-income countries. The World Bank, in particular, has been criticized for the weighted decision-making power given to its governors. The G8 and even G20, for example, are seen by other countries as a step back from a more democratic UN system. Others have drawn attention to the state-centric nature of GHG and the need to give a greater voice to non-state actors. In 1998, a delegation of the People's Health Assembly (PHA), a coalition of civil society organizations (CSOs) formed in 2000, met with incoming WHO Director-General Brundtland. Promising to give CSOs a greater voice within the organization, she fast-tracked official recognition of selected organizations to enable them to participate in FCTC negotiations (Collin et al. 2002). She also created an initiative to build closer links with CSOs. Progress since the late 1990s, however, has been disappointingly slow and CSOs have complained that private companies rather than civil society gained entry to the WHO under Brundtland. There was little progress under the short-lived tenure of Director-General Lee.

Over the past decade, the PHA has continued to call for the democratization of global health, publishing two editions of the *Global Health Watch* in an effort to hold global health initiatives to greater account. In 2010, the PHA launched the Democratizing Global Health Governance Project which seeks to reform the domination of GHG by major donor countries (namely, the US and European countries) and transnational pharmaceutical corporations which, it is argued, operate through the UN system, the Bretton Woods institutions, bilateral and regional trade agreements, bilateral aid and a slew of global public–private partnerships. WHO Watch is a subproject committed to 'the urgent reform of the forces and structures which shape global decision making and which affect the global health crisis and the right to health'.[7] With the aim of 'building capacity in supporting the WHO to regain its leadership role in global health governance', WHO Watch sent a letter to the 68th WHA offering comments on agenda items traditionally debated by states alone.[8] CSOs have also been critical of unaccountable entities such as charitable foundations (Eisenberg 2011), although equally some CSOs are themselves vulnerable to criticism of a lack of transparency and accountability. As argued by the PHA, 'the operating paradigm of this regime is strongly influenced by the ideology of neo-liberalism which is promoted through a much wider range of channels including the commercial media and various corporate peak bodies (such as at the World Economic Forum)'. In response, WHO Director-General Chan

TABLE 5.1 Representation in the plenary bodies of major global health initiatives

Institution	Plenary body	Membership
WHO	World Health Assembly	Delegations (led by Minister of Health) of 192 member states which each hold one vote in decision making
World Bank	Board of Governors	Governors (Ministers of Finance) appointed by 187 member countries, who hold decision-making power based on shares of World Bank stock held
UNICEF	Board of Directors	Mixture of donor and recipient countries
UNAIDS	Executive Cabinet	Executive Director, the Deputy Executive Directors of the Programme branch and the Management and External Relations branch, and the Director of the Executive Office
Global Fund to Fight HIV/AIDS, Tuberculosis and Malaria	Global Fund Board	Representatives from donor and recipient governments, civil society, the private sector, private foundations, and communities living with and affected by the diseases
Bill and Melinda Gates Foundation	Management Committee and Leadership Teams	Bill Gates, Melinda Gates, Bill Gates Sr., Warren Buffett and eight appointed individuals
Wellcome Trust	Board of Governors	Ten appointed individuals from the corporate sector and academia
PEPFAR	Office of the US Global AIDS Coordinator	Appointed head (ambassador)
UNITAID	Executive Board	One representative nominated from each of the five founding countries (Brazil, Chile, France, Norway and the UK), and Spain; One representative of African countries designated by the African Union; One representative of Asian countries; Two representatives of relevant civil society networks (nongovernmental organizations and communities living with HIV/AIDS, malaria or tuberculosis); One representative of the constituency of foundations; and One representative of the World Health Organization.

announced the need for renewed stakeholder engagement in 2010 as part of her reform agenda:

> WHO can bring people together. But when it comes to our own governance, we are, basically, an exclusive club. Our Constitution is a good one, but it limits decision-making to Member States. Our procedures for setting the agenda for international health work and defining policies and strategies do not give a voice to many others who have demonstrated their ability to have a decisive impact on health. I am referring to civil society organizations, global health initiatives, foundations, the private sector, industry, and many more. The challenge for WHO is to become more inclusive. (Chan 2011)

The Joint Action and Learning Initiative on National and Global Responsibilities for Health (JALI) was launched in 2010 by a 'coalition of civil society and academics, with a shared vision of the 'right of everyone to the enjoyment of the highest attainable standard of physical and mental health'. It argued that, above all, there was a need for 'fair and effective global governance for health – the organization of national and global norms, institutions, and processes that collectively shape the health of the world's population' (Gostin et al. 2010).

Institutionalization on Steroids: GHG amid Competing Normative Frameworks

The diverse and contested normative frameworks described above have produced a multitude of contrasting, often competing, global health initiatives. Indeed, the rapid proliferation of institutions since the 1990s, described as concerned with global health, has been a defining feature of GHG. Within donor countries, this is readily apparent. In the US, for example, there are seven executive branch departments, four independent or quasi-independent federal agencies, numerous departmental agencies/operating units, and several large-scale, multi-agency initiatives that comprise the government's 'global health architecture' (see figure 5.3). In addition, more than fifteen Congressional committees have jurisdiction and oversight over global health programmes, particularly those governing foreign assistance. Mirroring the global level, 'there is currently no formal, authoritative, coordinating mechanism for the US response' (Kates et al. 2009: 2). A similar situation can be found in other major donor countries such as Japan (Pilcavage forthcoming) and more recent donors such as Arab countries (Neumayer 2004) and China (Freeman and Boynton 2011).

At the global level, institutional growth can be mapped in a variety of ways. First, there have been initiatives created to focus on specific

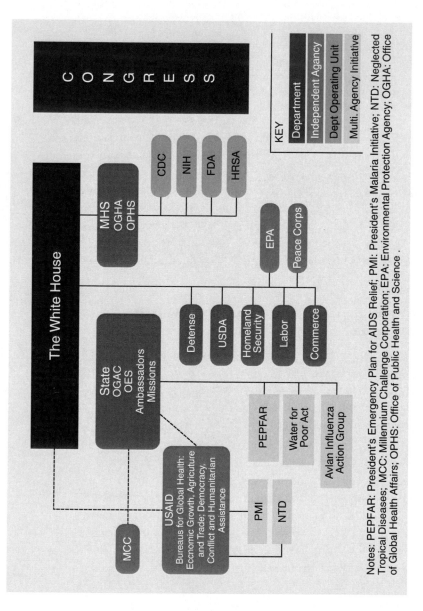

Notes: PEPFAR: President's Emergency Plan for AIDS Relief; PMI: President's Malaria Initiative; NTD: Neglected Tropical Diseases; MCC: Millennium Challenge Corporation; EPA: Environmental Protection Agency; OGHA: Office of Global Health Affairs; OPHS: Office of Public Health and Science .

Source: Kaiser Family Foundation (2011). Reprinted with permission from the Henry J. Kaiser Family Foundation.[9]

Figure 5.3 *Schematic of the US Government's Global Health Architecture*

disease areas. The largest number has been concerned with HIV/AIDS including UNAIDS, PEPFAR, International AIDS Vaccine Initiative (IAVI) and the World Bank Multi-country AIDS Programme (MAP) (Berstein and Sessions 2007). Other institutions, such as the GFATM, Drugs for Neglected Diseases Initiative (DNDi) and Global Council on Water Diseases, address multiple diseases. The Non-Communicable Disease Alliance, launched in 2009, represents 880 societies in 170 countries led by the International Diabetes Federation, Union for International Cancer Control, World Heart Foundation and the International Union against Tuberculosis and Lung Disease (IUATLD). Second, global health initiatives may support specific inputs or behaviours such as handwashing (Public–Private Partnership for Handwashing with Soap (PPPHW)), health systems strengthening (Global Health Workforce Alliance) and health information systems (Health Metrics Network). The GAVI Alliance was created to increase access to immunization in the world's poorest countries. PATH (Program for Appropriate Technology in Health) is an international non-profit organization seeking to improve global health by advancing technologies, strengthening systems and encouraging healthy behaviours.

Third, global health initiatives may be categorized by specific function. UNITAID, the International Financing Facility for Immunization (IFFIm) and Pneumococcal AMC (advanced market commitment) are innovative financing mechanisms. The Global Health Council has become an important advocacy group which aims to serve 'as the voice for action on global health issues and the voice for progress in the global health field' (Global Health Council no date). A large number of patient-driven foundations have been created to advocate for increased research and drug development for specific conditions such as the Global Network for Neglected Tropical Diseases and Global Network of People Living with HIV/AIDS. Product development partnerships, such as the Foundation for Innovative New Diagnostics (FIND), Malaria Vaccine Initiative and IAVI, focus on developing new technologies to address priority health needs in developing countries (Grace 2010; IAVI 2010). Fourth, global health initiatives can be characterized by their membership and governance. State-based global health-related institutions include WHO, UNICEF and other UN bodies, and the World Bank. Major non-state actors consist of charitable foundations, such as the Gates Foundation, Wellcome Trust and Rockefeller Foundation; nongovernmental organizations such as Save the Children Fund and Oxfam; and private corporations such as pharmaceutical and food companies. And, as if the numerous state and non-state institutions in global health were not confusing enough, some have combined to form hybrid organizations with public and private membership. The GFATM Board is composed of representatives from donor and recipient governments, civil society, the private sector, private foundations, and communities living with and affected by the diseases. Dozens of global public–private partnerships, such as the African Program for Onchocerciasis Control (APOC), bring together governments, intergovernmental organizations, civil society organizations and the private sector to address a broad range of global health issues.

Overall, attempts to map the GHG 'architecture', or even components of it over time, have proven challenging (Carlson 2004; World Bank 2007). As WHO Director-General Chan describes in 2011, there have been 'truly stunning increases in the number of actors, agencies, and initiatives funding or implementing programmes for health development. The landscape of public health is crowded. Activities in some areas, in some countries, are frankly chaotic' (Chan 2011). The World Bank's 2007 health strategy goes further: 'never before has so much attention – or money – been devoted to improving the health of the world's poor'; but it warns that 'unless deficiencies in the global aid architecture are corrected and major reforms occur at the country level, the international community and countries themselves face a good chance of squandering this opportunity' (World Bank 2007: 1).

This crowded and complex configuration of institutions concerned with global health have led to criticisms of policy incoherence, with gaps and overlaps in the health needs and populations served, and even competing and counterproductive activities. The most profound impact is on the ground in low- and middle-income countries, where many initiatives seek to operate. While increased resources for health development are very welcome, the demands of managing so many uncoordinated initiatives create a serious burden on governments and communities (Spicer and Walsh 2011). An example of this proliferation of agencies is given in figure 5.4.

While there is widespread lament of this overabundance of independent global health initiatives, it is important to examine the explanations for why GHG has evolved in this way and, correspondingly, what should be done about it. Substantial attention has been paid to the weaknesses of individual institutions, notably the WHO and its leadership role as the UN specialized agency for health (Andresen 2002). Criticisms of the organization are now like a well-worn script – its pedant bureaucracy and lack of institutional nimbleness, political nepotism, limited financial resources, overly broad and unfocused mandate, and, above all, its inability to command authority. Some conclude that the WHO has left a governance vacuum which others have rushed to fill by creating new institutional mechanisms. While lip service is often

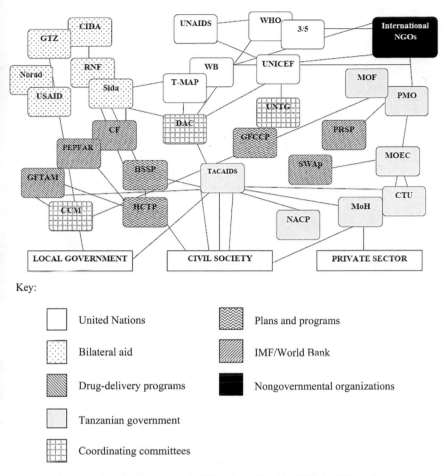

Key:

☐	United Nations	〰	Plans and programs
▦	Bilateral aid	▨	IMF/World Bank
▨	Drug-delivery programs	■	Nongovernmental organizations
☐	Tanzanian government		
▦	Coordinating committees		

Source: Jon Cohen (2006). 'The New World of Global Health', *Science*, 311 (5758), 166. Reprinted with permission from AAAS.

Figure 5.4 *Health initiatives related to HIV/AIDS operating in Tanzania in 2006*

paid to partnering with the WHO, in practice this constant institution building has served to undermine its capacity to be 'the world's health conscience'.

Where the core problem of GHG is seen as a lack of centralized authority, tasked with setting agreed priorities and allocating resources accordingly, there have been efforts to solve this issue with organizational or managerial remedies. This has been evident in the numerous attempts to create coordinating mechanisms based on the assumption that, with the right systems and structures in place, effective GHG can be achieved (table 5.2). The lead roles in each have varied, giving

TABLE 5.2 Initiatives to improve coordination in global health development assistance

Coordinating mechanism	Date	Lead role(s)	Activity
Donor consortia	1980s onwards	Aid agencies	Multiple aid donors pool resources for designated purpose and agree common procedures for reporting, monitoring and auditing
Sector-wide approach (SWAp)	Mid-1990s	Ministry of Health of aid recipient country	All significant funding to health sector to support single policy and expenditure programme under government leadership (Lucas 1998)
Millennium Development Goals	2000		Eight goals (including three health goals), with specific targets and indicators, that leaders of 189 UN member states agree to achieve by 2015
One Health Approach	2004		Manhattan Principles of twelve recommendations for establishing a more holistic approach to preventing epidemic/epizootic disease and for maintaining ecosystem integrity for the benefit of humans, their domesticated animals, and the foundational biodiversity that supports all life on Earth
Paris Declaration on Aid Effectiveness and Accra Agenda for Action	2005	OECD donor countries	A 'roadmap' to improve the quality of aid and its impact on development based on principles of ownership, alignment, harmonization, results and mutual accountability
Health 8	2007	WHO, UNICEF, UNFPA, UNAIDS, GFATM, GAVI, Gates Foundation, World Bank	Heads meet on a regular basis to review global health issues and discuss ways of aligning their work
International Health Partnership Plus (IHP+) Global Compact	2007	All governments, agencies and CSOs involved in improving health willing to sign up to commitments of IHP+	Improving health services and health outcomes by putting the Paris and Accra principles on aid effectiveness into practice
Multi-donor Secretariat for health MDGs	Proposed in 2007	Bilateral, multilateral institutions and foundations, global partnerships they fund, and	Framework for accountability and aid effectiveness for the initiative on 'Scaling Up for Better Health' (Anon. no date)

Name	Date	Actors	Description
Framework Convention on Global Health	Proposed in 2007	States, private sector and charitable sector	Legal instrument committing states to a set of targets, both economic and logistic, and to dismantle barriers to constructive engagement by the private and charitable sectors. It would stimulate creative public/private partnerships and actively engage civil society stakeholders. It could set achievable goals for global health spending; define areas of cost effective investment to meet basic survival needs; build sustainable health systems; and create incentives for scientific innovation for affordable vaccines and essential medicines (Gostin 2008)
Committee C of the World Health Assembly	Proposed in 2008	WHO	A committee to complement the work of Committee A (programme matters) and Committee B (budget and management) that would debate major health initiatives by other key players in the global health arena. It would provide the opportunity for these organizations to present their plans and achievements to the delegates of the WHA and the nongovernmental organizations in official relations with the WHO. It would also provide an opportunity to address coordination and common concerns of different partners in global health. Organizations wishing to make use of this mechanism would send their proposal to WHO's executive board, which would set the agenda for this committee as it does with the existing committees (Silberschmidt et al. 2008)
G8 Health Experts Group	2008	Group of Eight countries (US, Japan, Germany, UK, France, Russia, Canada, Italy)	An advisory group to the G8 which produces reports on the state of the world's health, principles for action, and proposed actions to be taken
Health Systems Funding Platform	2009	GAVI Alliance, GFATM, World Bank, WHO	Mechanism to accelerate progress towards the MDGs, and specifically to coordinate, mobilize, streamline and channel flow of existing and new international resources to support national health strategies

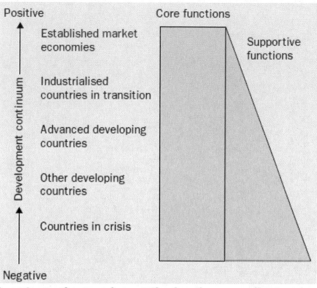

Importance of care and supportive functions according to economic circumstances

Source: Jamison et al. (1998: 515). Reprinted from *The Lancet*, Volume 351, Number 515, Jamison, Frenk and Knaul 'International collective action in health: objectives, functions and rationale', (1998) 514–17 with permission from Elsevier.

Figure 5.5 *The importance of core and supportive functions according to economic circumstances*

authority to coordinate respectively to donor agencies, recipient governments or the WHO. A related approach has been attempts to identify a rational division of labour among global health initiatives based on the comparative advantage of different players. A 1997 study of WHO's country-level activities, for example, eschew the traditional categories of *normative* and *technical* functions of the WHO, in favour of the term 'common global' and 'country specific' functions (Lucas 1998). Similarly, Jamison et al. distinguish between *core functions*, which 'transcend the sovereignty of any one nation state, and include promotion of international public goods (e.g., research and development), and surveillance and control of international externalities (e.g., environmental risks and spread of pathogens)'; and *supportive functions* which 'deal with problems that take place within individual countries, but which may justify collective action at international level owing to shortcomings in national health systems' (Jamison et al. 1998; see also figure 5.5). Certain global health institutions can fulfil different functions (e.g., the WHO serving core functions while the World Bank serves supportive functions). Ruger and Yach write that the WHO should achieve an optimal balance between a 'global role in advocacy, surveillance, standard setting, and research' and an 'operational work in specific countries and regions' (Ruger and Yach 2005: 1099–100). Reeves and Brundage identify the core strengths' of the WHO as public health surveillance, pandemic preparedness, and disaster response; global standard setting and regulation; catalysing global initiatives/partnerships for key health priorities; and advocating for policy change and behaviour change to combat noncommunicable diseases (Reeves and Brundage 2011).

Analysing the institutional dysfunction of GHG from a social constructivist perspective offers an alternative explanation. GHG, as it currently exists, is a product of the significant contestation among different normative frameworks defining global health problems and solutions. Thus, the diversity of institutions can be explained by the varied normative frameworks that have led to different, and sometimes competing, perspectives about the priority goals for global health and how to achieve them. From a security perspective, the US and other major donor countries can be observed as making funding decisions based on perceived national interests. 'Core' or 'common global' functions, as described above, have received support from major donor countries, while 'supportive' functions have been a harder sell. Another perspective which has led to the decline of the WHO has been the biomedically-based belief that the organization should focus on technical matters, based on medical science. This explains the disenchantment with the WHO from the 1970s, under Director-General Halfdan Mahler, who sought to challenge powerful vested interests, such as the pharmaceutical industry (Essential Drugs List), babyfood manufacturers (International Code on the Marketing of Breastmilk Substitutes), and launched the Health for All strategy. Criticism by the US government of these initiatives, as inappropriate politicization of the WHO, with health seen as a biomedical and technical field, was followed by the imposition of the policy of zero real growth in the WHO's budget in 1980. In the 1990s, the adoption of a policy of zero nominal growth reflected continued disenchantment with the WHO. In fine realist tradition, the US increasingly channelled its funding elsewhere, such as UNICEF. By the 2000s, it created its own global health initiatives led by PEPFAR and Global Health Initiative. The key feature of these arrangements is control.

The influence of normative frameworks is especially useful in explaining the proliferation of institutions concerned with HIV/AIDS. The creation of the Global Programme on AIDS (GPA) within the WHO reflected the initial desire to understand the biomedical aspects of the disease. The resistance by WHO Director-General Nakajima from the early 1990s to integrate a human rights perspective into the work of the GPA led to a falling out with its director, Jonathan Mann, and the eventual creation of UNAIDS with a broad approach to fighting the disease. A decade later, differences in perspective led to further institution building. US President Bush announced the creation of PEPFAR in 2003, with an initial US$15 billion of funding, despite the recent establishment of the GFATM. The Bush Administration's decision to channel the majority of its effort to fight HIV/AIDS bilaterally, rather than multilaterally, was criticized for creating yet more institutional structures and mechanisms. While the US government cited concerns with the GFATM's management of funding flows, the conservative interpretation of the ABC approach to HIV Prevention underpinning PEPFAR's work was an important factor (Dietrich 2007).

Conclusion

The 'chaotic' nature of GHG, as it exists in the early twenty-first century, is widely recognized as a fundamental hurdle to effective collective action. GHG, if it exists at all, is characterized by different layers and clusters of rule making and rule implementation authority, operating in many separate domains by disease area, activity area, function or membership. Despite recognition of the need for collective action, in short, there is little by way of global collectiveness. If governance is understood as a generally accepted set of formal and informal rules, norms and principles guiding members of a society in collective action for the purpose of achieving agreed goals, it can hardly be said that GHG exists at all. The multitude of institutional players populating the global health landscape, all convinced of the rightness of their mandates, and many determined to 'do their own thing', has created not only an anarchic system without a recognized central authority (Fidler 2006b), but one with multiple and competing worldviews and normative bases. Reform efforts now span decades, regularly focused on the weaknesses of the WHO and other individual institutions, as well as dysfunctions in the overall GHG system (or lack thereof). In this sense, Fidler's predictions of 'tectonic shifts' in GHG prompted by SARS and other global health threats, appear premature (Fidler 2004).

At the same time, it would be inaccurate to conclude that the current state of affairs in GHG is solely the result of realist self-interest and that, consequently, there is no collective spirit or action. This hardly explains the significant growth of health development assistance since the

1990s, despite the ups and downs of the world economy, quadrupling between 1990 and 2007 to US$22 billion per year. This does not account for the genuine efforts to fix the lack of leadership in GHG and to find answers to the 'too many cooks' conundrum. Nor does it recognize the growth of governance instruments adopted or proposed, some formal and others informal, to collectively regulate the global aspects of human health. Above all, it does not explain the remarkable outpouring of public and private support for global health causes, from record enrolments by students in training programmes to the boom in non-state initiatives, including charitable foundations, to improve global health.

There is no doubt that GHG is a complex and confusing landscape, highly flawed as an institutional base for collective action to tackle the broad array of issues comprising global health. It is right and proper that reflection and reform be undertaken with some urgency. However, this chapter has argued that how GHG has been problematized should form part of this reflection. Both the diagnosis of the shortcomings of GHG, as it currently exists, and visions of what GHG should be, cannot be separated from the numerous normative frameworks shaping global health thinking and practice. What we have is multiple visions of GHG resulting in both conflict and consensus. Few, if any, are presented as such. Instead, national interest (security), financial necessity (economism), scientific fact (evidence-based approach) or social complexity (social determinants of health), for example, are given as reasons for certain forms of GHG. Other normative frameworks, not covered in this chapter, can also be readily observed. Together, they have contributed to the creation of multiple multilateralisms, expressed through institutional forms that distribute power, authority and resources in different ways.

CHAPTER SIX
Security and Health

The link between security and health is not new, but has traditionally been seen in narrow terms largely relating to armed conflict. As the former WHO Director-General, Gro Harlem Brundtland explained:

> Historically in the West, disease was often seen as an impediment to exploration and a challenge to winning a war. Cholera and other diseases killed at least three times more soldiers in the Crimean War than did the actual conflict. Malaria, measles, mumps, smallpox and typhoid felled more combatants than did bullets in the American civil war. (Brundtland 2003: 417)

This early conceptualization of how health issues affect security is narrow, not only in the range of issues deemed as security threats (largely infectious diseases), but who is deemed at risk (namely armed forces). Traditional narratives also identify the manner in which conflict can affect health, both directly through casualties, as well as indirectly through, for example, its effects on health provision (such as the destruction of hospitals, fleeing of health workers, difficulties in the distribution of drugs) and the potential for refugees to spread disease. Thus, the impacts have been constructed in bi-directional, albeit narrow, terms: the manner in which disease may affect military capacity and especially military operations; and the impact of conflict on health and health care.

By the turn of the millennium, as Brundtland noted, these linkages were changing. A range of new issues had joined infectious disease as perceived security threats (see box 6.1), while concerns were no longer limited to the direct impacts on militaries and health provision, but also involved the wider effects on economic and political stability (Brundtland 2003: 421; see also WHO Europe 2007: 13). Furthermore, the salience of the linkages appeared to have increased. Within WHO, health security may have been first raised during Brundtland's tenure as Director-General, but interest grew into a major focus as reflected in the theme of the *World Health Report* and World Health Day of 2007 (WHO 2007a, 2007c). Nor was this interest confined to the WHO. The links between health and security were made by the UN Secretary General's *High Level Panel on Threats, Challenges and Change* in 2002, as part of its defining of a threat to international security as 'any event or process that leads to large-scale death or lessening of life chances' (UN High Level Panel 2004: 2). In January 2000, at its first meeting of the new millennium, the UN Security Council symbolically and significantly chose to discuss for the first time a health issue, HIV/AIDS (McInnes and Rushton 2010). The 2002 *US National Security Strategy*, coming in the immediate aftermath of the terrorist attacks of 11 September 2001 and the deliberate spread of anthrax shortly afterwards, elevated health to a security issue (White House 2002: 19). In the UK, pandemic influenza featured prominently in successive iterations of the national risk register and the UK *National Security Strategy* (Cabinet Office 2008: 14–15; Cabinet Office 2010: 27). Thus, in the first few years of the twenty-first century, a new narrative appeared which placed selected health issues higher on security agendas than ever before, while health agendas became far more sensitized to security concerns.

The rationale often cited for this new salience and broadened scope was constructed along fairly consistent lines: that new health risks had appeared as a result of emerging and re-emerging diseases, increased population mobility, spreading transnational crime, environmental change and bio-terrorism; and that these posed new security dangers (see, e.g., Brundtland 2003; WHO 2007a; Yuk-ping and Thomas 2010). Beyond 'real world' concerns, however, were political considerations, with some within the public health community recognizing that the

Box 6.1 World Health Day (2007) identification of international health security issues

To support the focus of the 2007 World Health Day on health security, the WHO produced a background document 'to help guide discussions and stir debate'. The paper identifies eight international health security issues. This list is worth highlighting because it encompasses most of the issues which feature in the debates on health security, although the list is perhaps longer than many others would identify and also reflects its origins in an international health organization.

Emerging diseases: new, highly contagious diseases, such as SARS and avian influenza, know no borders. Their potential to cause international harm means that outbreaks cannot be treated as purely national issues. In the last few decades, new diseases began emerging at an unprecedented rate of one or more per year.

Economic stability: public health dangers have economic as well as health consequences. Containing international threats is good for economic well-being. With fewer than 10,000 cases, SARS cost Asian countries US$60 billion of gross expenditure and business losses in the second quarter of 2003 alone.

International crises and humanitarian emergencies: these events kill and maim individuals and severely stress the health systems that people rely on for personal health security. In 2006, 134.6 million people were affected and 21,342 were killed by natural disasters.

Chemical, radioactive and biological terror threats: whether deliberate or accidental, WHO's global networks are well placed to respond to the health effects of these threats using the same techniques employed in other disasters – rapid assessment and response, triage and treatment, securing water, food and sanitation systems. Anthrax-tainted letters sent through the US postal system in 2001 and the release of sarin on the Tokyo subway in 1995 remind us that, although chemical and biological attacks are rare, there are people ready to use this brand of terrorism.

Environmental change: environmental and climate changes have a growing impact on health, but health policies alone cannot prevent their effects. People are dying – upwards of 60,000 in recent years in climate-related natural disasters, mainly in developing countries.

HIV/AIDS – a key health and security issue: the devastating impact of HIV/ AIDS, demonstrated to international security specialists the potential impact of a public health issue on security. In 2006, an estimated 39.5 million people were living with HIV/AIDS.

Building health security: national compliance with the revised IHR [International Health Regulations] 2005 will underpin international health security.

Strengthening health systems: functioning health systems are the bedrock of health security, but the current state of systems worldwide is inadequate. As an example, the world is currently short of more than four million health workers, with the impact most felt in developing countries. (WHO 2007c: 3)

security label was a potentially effective means of elevating health issues onto the national and global stages. In other words, constructing health as a security issue (i.e. 'securitized') could be seen as a pragmatic or strategic act to gain increased policy attention. Moreover, this was a period when security audiences had been sensitized to the idea of new risks following the 'bonfire of the certainties' at the end of the Cold War. The attempt to securitize health therefore fell on more fertile ground than might previously have been the case.

'Security', however, is not a straightforward concept. Indeed Barry Buzan has famously categorized it as 'essentially contested' – that is, a concept which generates unsolvable debates about its meaning and application (Buzan 1991: 7). This chapter identifies three broad meanings of health security: global health security (together with bio-security), human security, and national security. The purpose of this distinction is not simply heuristic but to suggest that each meaning is constructed for a particular purpose including promoting a certain agenda and privileging certain interests over others. This does not necessarily mean that different health issues occur with each meaning – some health issues are common, others are distinct. The key difference, rather, is whose interests are served and, in particular, what constitutes the referent object of health security. Whose security is being protected under each meaning? The object of this chapter, therefore, is not to identify some criteria whereby a health issue may or may not be considered a security issue. Instead, it is to reveal how health security, like other forms of security, is essentially contested and not amenable to a single set of agreed criteria, and thus reflects the interests and agendas of those constructing the concept.

Bio-security and Global Health Security

This section discusses two terms which have become increasingly prominent over the past decade. The first of these, 'bio-security', can be a somewhat vague term covering almost everything from national security threats arising from biological weapons to more general risks to public health. Part of the problem is that the term is used by commentators in a variety of different ways. Three in particular are worth highlighting. Some commentators (e.g., Enemark 2010) use it in a narrow and highly specific manner to discuss the risks posed by the development of new micro-organisms in science laboratories. These risks include both the deliberate and the inadvertent release of pathogens outside controlled laboratory environments. These scientific developments create a 'dual-use' dilemma:

> The tremendous advances in biology, biotechnology, genomics, proteomics, synthetic biology and bioinformatics in recent years are almost certain to lead to improved health and well-being through, for example, new diagnostics, treatments and vaccines to fight infectious diseases. Unfortunately, the possibility that a laboratory accident may lead to a major outbreak or that such advances may be deliberately misused to do harm on an unprecedented scale cannot be ignored. In other words, the knowledge and technologies that result from life science research used for legitimate research and technology development may also be appropriated for illegitimate intentions and applications (WHO 2007b: 1)

Box 6.2 identifies some of these dual-use dilemmas. As Christian Enemark (2010) points out, even trusted laboratory scientists may pose security risks: the main suspect of the US Federal Bureau of Investigation (FBI) for the release in 2001 of anthrax spores in letters addressed to US congressmen and the media was Bruce Ivins, a government scientist with high clearance levels who then committed suicide before his

Box 6.2 The dual-use dilemma

In 2007 a WHO working group identified three examples of 'research that has triggered concerns among scientists and the public':

Chemical synthesis of poliovirus cDNA

Researchers synthesized a poliovirus genome using chemically synthesized oligonucleotides and a map of the polio genome that was made publicly available on the internet. The result was a 'live' polio virus that paralysed mice. The paper that was published in *Science* in 2002 included a description of methods and materials. Concerns were raised that this provided a recipe that could be used to reconstruct the virus without obtaining a natural virus. One of the authors has stated: 'The widespread attention generated by our publication raised the overall awareness of the new reality of synthetic viruses and its possible consequences'.

Reconstruction of the 1918 flu virus

The successful reconstruction of the influenza A (H1N1) virus responsible for the 1918 'Spanish Flu' pandemic was published in *Science* and *Nature* in 2005. Some people raised concerns about the 'dangers of resurrecting the virus' and questioned whether the research should have been published. In its defence, the Centers for Disease Control and Prevention in the United States of America, one of the collaborators of the *Science* article, stated: 'While there are concerns that this approach could potentially be misused for purposes of bio-terrorism, there are also clear and significant potential benefits of sharing this information with the scientific community: namely, facilitating the development of effective interventions, thereby strengthening public health and national security'.

Inadvertently increasing the virulence of mousepox

In an attempt to control mice as pests, Australian scientists unexpectedly increased the virulence of mousepox. Their research, which was published by the *Journal of Virology* in 2001, was originally aimed at producing an infectious contraceptive for mice. By inserting a gene responsible for the production of interleukin-4 into the mousepox genome, the scientists created a pathogen that overcame the immune defence of mice and even killed mice that had been vaccinated. This unforeseen result and its publication raised the questions of whether the same technique could be applied to other orthopox viruses, such as smallpox, and what the consequences in terms of vaccination circumvention might be.

Source: WHO (2008a: 9).

arrest. As the numbers of laboratories and scientists involved increases, matched by increases in the numbers of biological agents and potential pathogens held in such locations, and in the movement of these pathogens internationally, so the risks appear to escalate.

Others use bio-security in a slightly different, but similarly specific, manner to refer to threats to national security from the deliberate use of pathogens, especially by terrorists (what is also called bio-terrorism and is discussed later in this chapter under 'National Security'. In contrast, others use it as a more generic term to cover a wide variety of possible health risks. Collier and Lakoff (2008), for example, identify four areas of bio-security risk: the appearance of new diseases such as SARS; bio-terrorism; the ability of fields such as synthetic biology to create new lethal organisms and the inadequacies of existing bio-safety protocols to deal with such developments; and food safety including both the contamination of the food supply (e.g., foot and mouth disease, vCJD, salmonella) and the risks involved in genetically modifying food sources. Although this list appears to concentrate on infectious diseases – whether natural or man-made, and whether inadvertently or deliberately released – its focus is clearly broader, as seen through the inclusion of genetically modified foodstuffs. This adds to the sense of vagueness over what bio-security refers to. One way around this is to identify two particular ways in which bio-security is used. The first focuses on those health issues which pose a risk to national security; and the second on those risks to health which have a global dimension. For the purposes of this chapter, the former are dealt with under the rubric of national security, and the second under global health security.

Although Steven Hoffman (2010) identifies four periods of global health security, each with their own distinct form of governance (see box 6.3), what these represent are phases of increasing *international* cooperation to protect *national* public health.

During the course of the first decade of the twenty-first century, however, the WHO (with others) increasingly changed the narrative to a more globalized view of health security. In 2002, for example, it explicitly linked health and security in arguing that the risks posed by infectious disease required a globalized response (WHO 2002), while later that decade it began work to address 'the risks and opportunities of life sciences research for global health security' (WHO 2007b: 3). The key moment, though, was the WHO's 2007 *World Health Report*, the sole focus of which was global public health security in the twenty-first century (WHO 2007a). In her introductory message to the report, WHO Director-General Margaret Chan wrote,

Box 6.3 Hoffman's Four Periods of Global Health Security Governance

Regime	Key characteristics
Unilateral quarantine regime (1377–1851)	• Disease causation unknown; Europe perceived as vulnerable to 'foreign diseases'. • Limited international cooperation; state sovereignty. • Fora for cooperation limited to few and infrequent sanitary councils.
Nascent sanitary conference regime (1851–92)	• Certain diseases recognized as contagious; Europe perceived as vulnerable to 'foreign diseases'. • Beginnings of international cooperation; state sovereignty. • Cooperation through conference diplomacy.
Institutionalized sanitary coordination regime (1892–1946)	• Broad acceptance of germ theory and of self-interest in disease eradication everywhere; Europe perceived as vulnerable to 'foreign diseases'. • International cooperation institutionalized; state sovereignty. • International sanitary conventions provide mechanism for cooperation.
Hegemonic health cooperation 1946–(C21?)	• Universal acceptance of germ theory; health as universal right. • Institutionalized international cooperation; state centricity. • International organizations for health promotion/ protection with powers to recommend state action.

Source: Hoffman (2010), especially p. 512 as adapted by the authors.

[health] threats have become a much larger menace in a world characterized by high mobility, economic interdependence and electronic interconnectedness. Traditional defences at national borders cannot protect against the invasion of a disease or vector. Real time news allows panic to spread with equal ease. Shocks to health reverberate as shocks to economies and business continuity in areas well beyond the affected site. Vulnerability is universal. (WHO 2007a: vi)

Although a number of states had already begun to identify global health issues as posing problems for their national security (including the UK, US and Australia), the WHO as an international body appeared to be casting the net wider. For WHO, health security appeared to be a world-wide problem where vulnerability was not national but 'universal'. This is seen in its understanding of what global health security is (see box 6.4). But what is also clear from WHO's use of the term, and in its use by other commentators (e.g., Baker and Forsyth 2007; Rodier 2007), is that what is meant by global health security is global threats to public

Box 6.4 WHO and global public health security

In its 2007 World Health Report, WHO discussed its understanding of global (public) health security in the following way:

> Public health security is defined as the activities required, both proactive and reactive, to minimize vulnerability to acute public health events that endanger the collective health of national populations.
>
> Global public health security widens this definition to include acute public health events that endanger the collective health of populations living across geographical regions and international boundaries. As illustrated in this report, global health security, or lack of it, may also have an impact on economic or political stability, trade, tourism, access to goods and services and, if they occur repeatedly, on demographic stability. Global public health security embraces a wide range of complex and daunting issues, from the international stage to the individual household, including the health consequences of human behaviour, weather-related events and infectious diseases, and natural catastrophes and man-made disasters, all of which are discussed in this report. (WHO 2007a: 1)

health security. Indeed chapter 2 of WHO's 2007 report on global health security is explicit in identifying 'threats to public health security'. In other words, what the WHO is primarily interested in here is how risks to public health have been globalized, and not so much in how global public health risks affect the broader security interests of individuals or states. In this sense, its focus appears different from the other two meanings discussed in this chapter, (inter-)national and human security, although it does acknowledge that risks exist to broader security concerns, principally economic security. Nevertheless, the subject of global health security is not security but health.

In its discussion of global health security, the WHO structures its report into three broad categories of risks (WHO 2007a: iii–iv):

- *existing threats* to public health security, including inadequate investment in public health, conflict-induced public health crises, microbial change, antibiotic resistance, infectious disease, animal husbandry and food-processing, environmental change and accidents involving toxic chemicals (including radioactive events);
- *new threats* which have emerged in the twenty-first century, specifically bio-terrorism, new infectious diseases such as SARS and the dumping of toxic chemicals;
- and *threats which are on the horizon*, including pandemic influenza, extensively drug-resistant TB and polio.

In so doing, the report suggests that, not only has globalization added new dimensions to these longstanding problems, but that new risks are emerging, some of which can be identified but implicitly others may not be. What is also clear is that, although the focus of the report shares much in common with Collier and Lakoff's understanding of bio-security – concerns over infectious disease, food safety and bio-terrorism – global health security is conceived in even broader terms. Included in the WHO's understanding of global health security, for example, is a much greater interest in industrial concerns (the health implications of chemical and radiological accidents, and the dumping of toxic waste) as well as concerns over the impact of natural disasters and environmental change. As a result, the WHO's presentation of global heath security may be placed into three main, if somewhat broad, categories of risk. The first is infectious disease, motivated not so much by the continued existence of diseases, such as malaria, which are endemic to large parts of the world, but by new diseases or new variants of known diseases which pose new risks and hazards. The second is food safety, especially risks arising from the industrialization of agriculture exacerbated by the global nature of the food industry, as seen, for example, in the 2011 outbreak of *E. coli* in Germany. The third are catastrophes affecting the natural environment, whether deliberate, accidental or natural in origin. These include industrial accidents, such as toxic spills, the dumping of chemicals, and nuclear incidents such as Chernobyl and Fukushima; the release of pathogens through breaches of laboratory safety protocols or their deliberate use by terrorists; and extreme natural events (albeit some of which may be anthropogenic), such as the European heatwave in 2003 or the Japanese earthquake and tsunami of 2011.

What is also clear is that, from the WHO's perspective, global health security is a call for action. Its analysis of global health risks leads to a very clear prescription to develop 'collective international public health action [to] build a safer future for humanity' (WHO 2007a: ix; see also Wilson et al. 2008: 48). Indeed the WHO *defines* global health security in terms of actions:

> global health security is defined as the activities required, both proactive and reactive, to minimize vulnerability to acute public health events that endanger the collective health of populations living across geographical regions and international boundaries. (WHO 2007a: ix)

Typical of the sort of collaborative action envisaged under global health security are the revised International Health Regulations (IHRs) of 2005 which became binding international law for 193 signatories in

2007. The fact that these regulations were finally agreed two years after the SARS epidemic was almost certainly not coincidental – they were driven by an increased awareness of new global health threats and the necessity to develop more effective surveillance and control practices. The new IHRs required states to establish mechanisms to detect, assess, notify and report public health events of international concern, and thereby protect against the spread of public health emergencies. What is interesting, however, is the manner in which this long-established public health instrument was explicitly linked to global health security. Wilson et al. (2008: 44) refer to the IHR (2005) as 'a major step forward in protecting global health security', while Baker and Forsyth (2007) describe them as 'a revolutionary change in global health security'. In an interview in the *Bulletin of the World Health Organization*, the WHO's Director of IHR coordination, Guenael Rodier, stated that 'In the IHR, public health overlaps with national security' (Rodier 2007: 429), while in a co-authored article published the same year, he describes the IHRs as 'a key driver in the effort to strengthen global public health security' (Rodier et al. 2007: 1447). Significantly, one of Rodier's co-authors in the latter piece was David Heymann, author of the 2007 *World Health Report*, which advanced the idea of global health security. Heymann went on to become Director of the Centre on Global Health Security, Chatham House in 2009.

This prescriptive dimension can also be seen in some of the literature on bio-security. Collier and Lakoff (2008: 7), for example, talk of bio-security as an attempt to bring together previously distinct fields of health and politics to effect change. Fidler writes of the emergence of bio-security as a 'transformational moment' in public health as a governance activity (Fidler 2006a: 196; see also Fidler and Gostin 2008). Because of this, the use of the term 'security' begins to appear less as an analytical tool, and more as a strategic or pragmatic practice. In other words, the term is used not to describe a condition but to increase awareness and encourage action for change by adding a sense of urgency and importance. Of course, there is nothing new in using security in this manner, and the use of the term in this way does not necessarily invalidate it. Vuori (2008), for example, discusses how use of the word 'security' can be a 'claim speech act', used to raise an issue on decision makers' agendas. Thierry Balzacq (2005: 172) similarly argues that it can be used as a strategic or pragmatic practice to encourage action. Accepting the position of Vuori and Balzacq then leads to an understanding of global health security, not as an objective condition, but as something constructed by someone and for some purpose. From this perspective, global health is not a security issue because it meets independent conditions or criteria for security, but because it has been labelled so by an authoritative actor able to convince its audience (see Buzan et al. 1997) and, in this instance, to gain attention and develop action. But this then raises the question of for what purpose? And the answer is quite clear: improved health on a global scale. Global health security, therefore, is not about the security or stability of the state or any other collective grouping. Rather, it is about promoting health, a traditional task of health services nationally but now taken by the WHO onto a global stage with added urgency.

Human Security

Although the philosophical roots of human security lie deeply embedded in classical liberalism's emphasis upon the individual, like biosecurity and global health security, human security is a relatively new concept. In 1990 Mahbub ul-Haq launched the first annual report from the United Nations Development Programme (UNDP), the *Human Development Report*, arguing that development should be based not on states but on people; not just on economic well-being but on health, education and basic freedoms; and that security was more than the protection of national boundaries (UNDP 1990; see also ul-Haq 1995). This approach was further developed in the UNDP's 1994 *Human Development Report* which focused on human security and is often seen as the originator of the concept. In this latter report, it was argued that security

> has for too long been interpreted narrowly: as security of territory from external aggression, or as protection of national interests in foreign policy . . . Forgotten were the legitimate concerns of ordinary people who sought security in their daily lives . . . For many of them, security symbolized protection from the threat of disease, hunger, unemployment, crime, social conflict, political repression and environmental hazards . . . For most people, a feeling of insecurity arises more from worries about daily life than from the dread of a cataclysmic world event. (UNDP 1994: 22)

Health security was explicitly identified as a component of human security (e.g., UNDP 1994: 24) and health in general, but disease in particular runs through the 1994 report as a threat to human security. Significantly, the report came at a time when humanitarian crises in Rwanda and the former Yugoslavia were high on the international agenda, and where protection of the vulnerable was perceived to be a global responsibility. Moreover, such crises were described as 'complex' – that is, they were not simply military but multi-dimensional in nature, requiring a response which encompassed multiple fields including education and health care.

By the turn of the millennium, human security was receiving considerable attention, not least because of the efforts of a small number of key advocates including then Canadian Minister of Foreign Affairs Lloyd Axworthy (1997, 2001), Nobel laureate Amartya Sen (Sen 2000), and academics Lincoln Chen and Caroline Thomas (Thomas, 2000; Chen at al. 2003; Chen 2004). The highpoint perhaps came in 2003 with the report of the Commission on Human Security, an initiative supported by UN Secretary-General Kofi Annan and chaired by Sen and former UN High Commissioner for Refugees Sadako Ogata (Ogata and Sen 2003). In this report, Ogata and Sen reiterated the view of human security which had been developing since the UNDP's 1994 report, that human security was about freedom from want, freedom from fear, and the capacity of individuals to take action on their own behalf:

> Human security is concerned with safeguarding and expanding people's vital freedoms. It requires both shielding people from acute threats and empowering people to take charge of their own lives . . . Human security naturally connects several kinds of freedom – such as freedom from want and freedom from fear, as well as freedom to take action on one's own behalf. (Ogata and Sen 2003: iv and 10)[1]

Human security is strongly linked to the promotion of human rights, often explicitly so (e.g., Ogata and Cels 2003: 274). It is also emancipatory in its aim, in that it attempts to free people whether from fear, want or other forms of oppression. And running through it is a strong and often explicit normative bias – that the world can and should be run in a different, better way by putting people first.

At the heart of human security is the simple but – in security terms at least – radical idea that *people matter*. The focus of security is shifted from the state to people, either as individuals or as communities. As Axworthy explains:

> Security has traditionally focused on the state because its fundamental purpose is to protect its citizens. Hobbled by economic adversity, outrun by globalization, and undermined from within by bad governance, the capacity of some states to provide this protection has increasingly come into question . . . The state has, at times, come to be a major threat to its population's rights and welfare . . . This drives us to broaden the focus of security beyond the level of the state and toward individual human beings, as well as to consider appropriate roles for the international system to compensate for state failure . . . This shift reflects a growing recognition that the protection of people must be a principal concern. (Axworthy 2001: 19).

Thus human security stands in contrast to state security: whereas the latter focuses on the preservation of the state and its institutions, human security is concerned with risks to individuals. In general, however, most advocates of human security do not see it as replacing but rather complementing state security. Indeed, a stable state may be a prerequisite for human security. Ogata and Cels, for example, write that 'State security is essential but does not necessarily ensure the safety of individuals and communities . . . Human security thus shifts attention from securing states to protecting peoples within and across state borders. In so doing, it reinforces the assertion of sovereignty as a responsibility' (Ogata and Cels 2003: 275). Thus human security *expands on* rather than replaces the idea of security as threats to the state, covering those risks and actors which threaten individuals and communities, and including the idea of 'empowering people to fend for themselves' (Ogata and Sen 2003: 4). Indeed, Ogata and Cels even suggest that 'Under certain conditions state security can take precedence over human security interests' (Ogata and Cels 2003: 275).

Human security, however, is more than simply putting people first and expanding the security agenda to accommodate risks to individuals and communities. Rather, it portrays the world as turbulent and insecure even when there is peace. It differs in this way from national security's highly structured view of insecurity as militarized violence, with its emphasis upon formal actors (mainly states), defined tools (largely military, economic and diplomatic power), and a tendency towards a binary divide between peace (security) and war (insecurity). For human security, risks are much less certain and rather more complex, arising from both the interconnectedness and multiplicity of types of risks that individuals may face. Mark Duffield describes it as 'the difference between seeing the world as a machine and seeing it as a living system or organism . . . [of moving] from the study of objects to the study of interconnections' (Duffield 2001: 9–10). Running through the human security approach, therefore, is a sense that the world has changed through globalization and that the state can no longer always mediate successfully between the individual and these new global forces. The links with development are also clear, not only in the origins of the human security approach with the UNDP, but also the shared concern with how lives are lived. But, whereas development is about improving the quality of human life, human security is concerned with the risks to life and the freedom to live life without fear (Ogata and Sen 2003: 10).

That health is a human security issue appears unchallenged. To some extent, this is because health fits into human security's view of the emergence of transnational threats which states are no longer able to mediate but which affect the lives of individuals (Curley and Thomas 2004: 19–20). In particular, potentially epidemic infectious disease seems to fit the mould of a human security issue, given the construction of it as a new risk and one which can transcend borders (Ogata and Sen 2003: 97; Curley and Thomas 2004: 20). Not all health issues are cast as threats to human security, however. In an attempt to identify what was and was not a health security issue, the Commission on Human Security suggested four criteria (see box 6.5), which appear to be more prescriptive than analytical. Lincoln Chen, a member of the Commission, offers a different take on the linkage:

> Health and security are tightly linked. Good health is 'intrinsic' to human security, since human survival and good health are the core of 'security'. Health is also 'instrumental' to human security because good health enables the full range of human functioning. (Chen 2004: 2)

More commonly, commentators have tended to focus on two of human security's key freedoms: freedom from want (to some extent implied in Chen's 'full range of human functioning') and freedom from fear (to some extent Chen's 'human survival'). On the former, the link is not only about the manner in which health is fundamental to an individual's quality of life and dignity; it is also, and more importantly, about the relationship between health and poverty (Ogata and Cels 2003: especially 278–9). This relationship may be characterized as a feedback loop: poverty leads to poor health, which in turn increases levels of poverty. But improved health may lead to rises in living standards as well as a better quality of life as people become better able to work and less dependent upon health services (see, e.g., WHO 2001). The political salience of this relationship increased in the years after the millennium. The war on poverty became a rallying cry not only for development activists, but also among key international institutions such as the World Bank and major donor countries, especially the G8 at the 2005 Gleneagles summit. These same global players also committed themselves to improving health worldwide, through the MDGs and the establishment of the Global Fund.[2] That these efforts came at the same time as the idea of human security was gathering momentum, with the Commission on Human Security reporting in 2003, seemed more than serendipitous, and even suggested a humanitarian *zeitgeist*. There was an additional reason why health was an important element in human security and especially in reducing fear from want. It not only contributed directly to an individual's quality of life, but to the economic life of a state. As Gro Harlem Brundtland argued, there was

> **Box 6.5 What makes a health issue a human security risk?**
>
> In its Report, the Commission on Human Security identify four criteria that influence the strength of links between health and human security:
>
> - The scale of the disease burden now and into the future.
> - The urgency for action.
> - The depth and extent of the impact on society.
> - The interdependencies or 'externalities' that can exert ripple effects beyond particular diseases, persons or locations.
>
> Source: Ogata and Sen (2003: 97).

a need to invest in health as 'a prerequisite for economic development and an important part of any development strategy' (Brundtland 2003: 421). A generally good standard of health among the population was constructed by, for example, the WHO Commission on Macroeconomics and Health (WHO 2001) as a key factor in economic stability and development which, in turn, would feed back into individual security through reduced fears over health and economic survival.

Health also contributed significantly to the second of human security's key freedoms – the freedom from fear. Interestingly this was not so much constructed in terms of fear of disease or other health risks, but rather in the more traditional terms of state stability and military security (e.g., Brower and Chalk 2003: 8–9; Ogata and Sen 2003: 97; Chen 2004: 4–5). Three concerns are commonly raised. First, health crises may affect confidence in a state and the social order. If the state's duty is to protect its citizens, but it is failing to do so from health threats, then the social contract between the state and the governed is broken. This is especially so if disparities in health care are exacerbated by social divisions such as socioeconomic class, ethnic grouping or regional identity: when some groups receive better health care because of who they are rather than because of what they need. Health crises may also affect regional stability if they prompt population movements, either due to large-scale migration or the spread of disease via migration. Finally military security may be affected by health crises. Troops have historically been more at risk from disease than from the battlefield and, although antibiotics and better health care in theatres of war have altered this for many armed forces, troops remain more vulnerable, including a higher incidence of sexually transmitted diseases (e.g., HIV/AIDS).[3]

How valid some of these concerns are as security risks, however, is debatable. For example, there is no evidence that health crises can act

Box 6.6 Mixing human and national security in health

Speaking on 'AIDS and Global Security' to a Nobel Centenary Roundtable in 2002, WHO Director-General Gro Harlem Brundtland revealed the manner in which human and national security could be elided.

> What is emerging today is a notion of 'human security'. The levels of ill health in countries constituting the majority of the world's population pose a direct threat to their own national economic and political viability, and therefore to the global economic and political interests of all countries . . . So investing in global health is investing in national security. (Brundtland 2002)

as anything more than a contributory factor affecting confidence in the state (as opposed to confidence in a particular government). Migration appears to be more a function of a lack of other basic needs, including food and clean water, than health care. And although historically the impact of disease on military performance has had potentially a major impact on state security (for example, English King Henry V risked defeat by the French, and the collapse of Plantagenet rule at Agincourt, because his forces had been severely depleted by dysentery during the siege of Harfleur in 1415), the link today is much weaker. This suggests that the power of the argument is derived from something other than its basis in a perceived empirical reality. What this move, linking freedom from fear to issues such as state stability, does accomplish is to help blur the difference between human and national security (see, for example, box 6.6). That human security's emphasis on freedom from fear overlaps with national security leads to the potential for confusion and misunderstanding.

Despite the interest generated in human security in some quarters, and its apparent complementarities with the increased interest in humanitarianism and poverty relief at the turn of the millennium, human security has failed to shake the dominance of national security as the dominant paradigm. To a significant extent, this may be due to the manner in which Western governments have been able to construct terrorism both as the dominant security concern after 9/11 and as a national security problem. This, in turn, suggests the continued power of states, especially Western states, to construct security narratives in spite of human security's emphasis on states being as much the problem as the solution, and the inability of states to deal with new risks. Yet it is also, to some extent, the product of human security's vagueness as a concept. As Roland Paris comments, everyone is for it, but few people have a clear idea of what it means . . . [definitions] tend to be extraordinarily expansive and vague, encompassing everything from physical security to psychological well-being, which provides policymakers with little guidance in the prioritization of competing policy goals (Paris 2001: 88)

For critics such as Paris, human security is 'slippery by design' (2001: 88), a concept which is kept deliberately vague to ensure maximum support from diverse constituencies, but which then makes it ultimately little more than a slogan. In its all-encompassing nature, it becomes difficult to see what, if anything, is excluded from human security, and therefore it has limited analytical or policy value. Moreover, in its expansive articulation of security as encompassing social, economic and cultural well-being, it becomes difficult to see the difference between cause and effect: the causes of insecurity (poverty, poor health, economic deprivation) are also the effects of insecurity (Paris 2001: 93). As a consequence, human security has not had the impact in both policy and academic circles which its proponents had hoped for.

National and International Security

National security is often characterized in a narrow manner: that the referent object of security is the state; that the main concerns are direct threats, usually military in nature; and that the context is one of an anarchic international states system where self-help is the order of the day. Security therefore depends on the state protecting itself from such threats, and a social contract is entered into whereby citizens forsake some of their individual freedoms (in the most extreme form through conscription in time of war) to secure the greater collective good. The risk, however, is that the social contract is undermined by the increasing power of the state, which may view its own preservation more highly than the lives and lifestyles of its citizens. The state, therefore, may become willing to sacrifice the freedoms and rights of the people it is supposed to protect in order to preserve its own power. It is this fear that has led to many health practitioners – ostensibly concerned with protecting and promoting the well-being of individuals and communities – to be wary of national security.

This characterization, however, is more of a caricature than an accurate reflection of contemporary thinking on national security in three ways. First, this characterization is overly restrictive in its understanding of how national security is practised. Even if military threats are the only direct risks to state survival, military strength depends on other factors, not least economic power and social coherence. Therefore, policies other than military can have a major effect on state security. Few states, moreover, can rely solely on their own strengths for security, entering instead into security communities or formal alliances whereby some independence is traded for mutual support (hence in part the development of the term 'international security', although often national and international are used interchangeably). Second, for more than two decades, in the West at least, national security's traditional focus on military threats has been replaced by a more diverse range of risks. This broadening of the security agenda has created a space where issues such as health can be considered part of national security. But it has also created the attendant question of what *is* a security issue? As a result, the new boundaries of security can appear so vague as to make the question what is *not* a security issue more pertinent. Crucially, failure to satisfactorily define what is (and what is not) a security issue has risked turning 'security' into an empty signifier, a term readily applicable to any issue, and therefore devoid of substantive meaning. This has led some to argue for a return to a more restrictive definition (see Deudney 1990; Walt 1991; Freedman 1998: 53), although most accept that national security in the twenty-first century is far more than defence of territorial integrity from a military threat. Third, although the focus on states remains, understandings of the state and state power have changed. Of particular significance for health security is the shift away from sovereign power and towards governmentality. Drawing on the work of French philosopher Michel Foucault, both Stefan Elbe and Alan Ingram have argued that power is no longer oriented self-referentially towards preserving the power of the state (sovereign power) but rather towards improving the welfare of citizens (governmentality). Ingram cites Foucault: 'What can the end of government be? Certainly not just to govern, but to improve the condition of the population, to increase its wealth, its longevity *and its health*' (quoted in Ingram 2010: 608, emphasis added; see also Elbe 2009: 86–107). Of course, this is not the case for all states, and both Elbe and Ingram accept that it applies predominantly to Western states; but as these states have set the agenda for health security, the significance of this shift is considerable.

National security's interest in health has been longstanding in that the physical condition of military troops affects their operational performance. As noted above, diseases such as cholera and dysentery have historically caused significant numbers of casualties during military campaigns. From the 1990s on, however, interest in a broader range of concerns began to develop and started to become apparent within a number of key policy circles. In so doing, the foreign and security policy community have maintained a robustly state-centric approach. In published statements by foreign and security ministries, there is consider-able consistency in prioritizing the national interest when discussing health security issues (e.g., Cook 2000: 2; Downer, 2003; FCO 2003: 13; US State Department 2004: 76). Two examples of this are the 1999 US National Intelligence Estimate on the global threat of infectious disease to the United States, and the January 2000 meeting of the UN Security Council. On the first, in 1999 the Central Intelligence Agency (CIA) identified a number of risks to US security arising from infectious disease, risks exacerbated by rapid globalization and the increased worldwide movement of goods and people. These included not only risks to US citizens travelling abroad, but to citizens at home given the potential for certain infectious diseases to spread globally. Crucially, however, the CIA went further than this, arguing that infectious disease also posed a risk to international stability and even economic growth, thus placing it firmly in the territory of national security (CIA 2000). On the second, at its first meeting of the new millennium, the UN Security Council discussed the threat of HIV/AIDS to Africa and, in Resolution 1308, warned 'that the HIV/AIDS pandemic, if unchecked, may pose a risk to stability and security' (UNSC 2000b; see also UNSC 2000a; McInnes and Rushton 2010). In particular, the Security Council drew attention to the effects of HIV/AIDS on social stability and on peacekeeping missions. This debate raised the global political stakes on HIV/AIDS and, in subsequent years, HIV/AIDS has been framed not only as a humanitarian catastrophe but as a risk to national security and international stability.

Three issues have dominated national security's interest in and engagement with health: acute and severe infectious diseases of epi-demic potential; HIV/AIDS; and bio-terrorism (see boxes 6.7, 6.8 and 6.9). What is missing, however, is a rationale as to why some health issues might be considered national security problems but not others. Health issues are not identified as national security risks by reference to an explicit set of criteria, but have rather arisen in an ad hoc manner and agreed inter-subjectively by key national and international actors. Although it is possible to identify three broad sets of reasons which suggest an implicit agenda, as will be seen below, these are also prob-lematic. The first of these reasons is the potential of a health issue to threaten international stability. Four possible reasons can, in turn, be identified as supporting this claim.

The first of these is that health crises may have dramatic effects on the global economy. That health crises may have detrimental economic effects has been long understood, but globalization has not only increased this sensitivity, but also broadened the potentially affected geographical territory. An epidemic may lead to reduced economic growth in areas not directly affected by the disease, or even in worst-case scenarios trigger a global recession, increasing levels of poverty and creating stresses on lifestyle and livelihood among even the wealthy states. Second, poverty and poor health may lead to migration as people seek a better, safer life elsewhere. It is feared that migration flows can not only risk spreading disease, but may act as destabilizing forces in a region. Third, it is argued that militaries may be at increased risk from some diseases, especially HIV/AIDS, impacting upon their operational capabilities with potential effects on national security and thereby international stability. Finally, risks from certain diseases (and in particular HIV/AIDS) are believed to affect the willingness of states to send troops on peacekeeping missions. Concerns have also been expressed at the willingness of countries to receive peacekeepers if they fear that troops may bring high rates of HIV infection into a country with them. The problem with these four arguments is that the causal relationship between an adverse health effect and international stability is questionable, and/or the empirical evidence to support the claim is suspect or missing. For example:

- On the macro-economic effects of poor health, the long-term sensitivity of the global economy to changes in health status are unclear while there is no credible evidence that international stability is affected by these effects. Neither sudden outbreak events such as SARS and pandemic influenza, nor chronic diseases such as malaria and (increasingly) HIV/AIDS, have affected international stability because of their macroeconomic effects; nor have SARS and pandemic influenza demonstrated significant long-term macroeconomic effects (although assessing the impact of the 2009 H1N1 influenza pandemic is complicated by the simultaneous global financial crisis).
- Although there is an awareness of migration as a security issue (see, e.g., Weiner 1992–3; Huysmans 1997; in contrast, see Graham and Poku 2000), health status does not appear to be a key driver in people leaving their homes. Rather, poverty, famine and conflict appear to be much more significant causes of mass migration.
- Although there was some evidence at the turn of the decade that militaries were more susceptible to HIV infection, and a number of plausible reasons were offered for this, the picture now appears more nuanced. Empirical evidence is no longer so clear cut, while HIV/AIDS awareness campaigns have been instituted (not least by UNAIDS) which have the potential to massively reduce HIV infection rates among military personnel (McInnes 2006, 2007; ASCI 2009).

- The link between a military weakened by disease and state instability/ insecurity is also unclear. Empirical evidence is lacking for this, while the literature on the causes of war remains contested over the issue of military weakness. The best that may be said is that, if insecurity emerges, then a weakened military may be less able to cope than one which has not been affected by poor health.
- Research during the last decade on the global spread of HIV/AIDS does not support the argument that peacekeeping is an important vector in the spread of the disease or that peacekeepers are especially susceptible (UNAIDS 2005; UN DPKO 2005).

Box 6.7 Infectious disease as a national security risk

Three broad reasons have been articulated by the foreign and security policy community as to why infectious disease is a national security risk. First, the spread of these diseases could pose a direct threat to the health and well-being of the very people that states are there to protect, including crucially, and for the first time in perhaps half a century, the populations of Western states. This is especially important in the context of the shift away from sovereign power and towards governmentality. Concerns were first articulated in the late 1990s, most notably by the CIA's 1999 National Intelligence Estimate on the threat from infectious disease. But it was the emergence of SARS in 2002–3 which did most to alert states to the fact that new diseases can spread quickly and uncontrollably, while in the middle of the decade the likelihood of pandemic flu and the possibility of a strain of H5N1 (avian flu) spreading from human to human posed the possibility of deaths from disease on a scale not witnessed in the industrialized world since the Spanish flu. These fears were given a touch of reality by the swine flu pandemic of 2009, not least by the way in which it spread widely and rapidly. The disease appeared to outstrip initial public health responses as well as place strains on the provision of drugs. Swine flu also demonstrated how such diseases could create public fears, partly related to the intense media interest which were perhaps disproportionate to the eventual levels of morbidity and mortality (especially when compared to endemic diseases such as malaria, or tobacco-related diseases). Perhaps ironically the intense media concern followed by a comparatively small number of deaths may have led some to believe that the risks of pandemic influenza had been overstated and contributed towards a sense of pandemic fatigue. Nevertheless, pandemic influenza continues to be considered a high risk by many western states.

Second, a pandemic may cause social disruption and threaten the stability of a state, especially one which is already weak: by eroding confidence in the state's ability to provide a basic level of protection against disease; social inequalities may be highlighted as the rich or privileged obtain access to better drugs or health care, potentially leading to public disorder; if large numbers of people die or are unwilling/unable to go to work, public services may be placed at risk, threatening the functioning of a state; and violence and disorder may appear if the authorities become unable to cope and if groups feel they have nothing to lose. Thus a state may begin to fail. Although disease may not be the sole cause, it may provide the tipping point, turning a 'weak state' into a 'failed' one. Moreover, this is not simply an issue for the state directly affected. As the United States' 2002 *National Security Strategy* put it, 'America [and the West] is threatened less by conquering states than we are by failing ones' (White House 2002: 1).

Third, a large-scale epidemic may also contribute to economic decline by: forcing increased government spending on health as a percentage of GDP; reducing productivity due to worker absenteeism and the loss of skilled personnel; reducing investment (internal and external) because of a lack of business confidence; and by raising insurance costs for health provision. For the state involved, the costs may be highly significant, but in a globalized world the effects may be felt much more widely. The relatively short-lived SARS outbreak of 2003–3 led to less than a thousand deaths – individually tragic but, compared to annual deaths from HIV/AIDS, TB or malaria, statistically relatively insignificant; but the loss in trade and investment was calculated in tens of billions of US dollars for the economies in Asia. The macroeconomic effects of a major epidemic may therefore be very significant, threatening to make the relatively affluent poor and the already poor poorer, with a consequent impact upon the ability of states and individuals to provide for their security and well-being.

Box 6.8 The case for HIV/AIDS as a national security issue

Although an infectious disease, HIV/AIDS is often constructed as a security issue in its own right. This status was both reflected in and reinforced by the UN Security Council's special session on HIV/AIDS in 2000, the Council's subsequent Resolution 1308 on the threat to Africa from the disease, and its reaffirmation of the link in 2011. The claims made in 2000 by the Security Council were decisive in constructing the agenda for the subsequent debate which emerged in the following few years on HIV/AIDS as a national security issue.

A number of concerns were regularly cited which included the effects of the disease on economies and on governance (e.g., ICG 2001; Justice Africa 2004). HIV/AIDS was claimed to create particularly severe economic problems because of the cumulative effects of the disease over a number of years and because of its disproportionate impact upon workers in what should be the most productive period of their lives (UN Secretariat 2003: xiii–xiv; ICG 2001: 9–13). Such economic decline may increase income inequalities and poverty, exacerbating or creating social and political unrest. HIV infection rates were seen as being unusually high among skilled professionals (including civil servants, teachers, police and health workers) and young adults, threatening 'the very fibre of what constitutes a nation' (ICG 2001: 1). Governance could be harmed if societies become polarized as a consequence of HIV/AIDS, if disaffection with the political process sets in, or as a consequence of aid-dependency. The stigma of AIDS may also lead to exclusion from work and/or society, creating alienation, fatalism and anger among people, especially young people, living with HIV and AIDS.

Continued

These people may become prone to criminal violence or to following violent leaders (CIA 2000; Justice Africa 2004).

The high rate of HIV infection among security forces, including the military, was also frequently cited as a cause for concern. This was a particular problem in sub-Saharan Africa, where infection rates among the military were reported to be especially high, with consequences for combat readiness, military performance, morale and defence budgets (as money is diverted to caring for HIV-positive military personnel). Because of this, states may be at greater risk from internal conflict or external aggression. Moreover, there was some evidence to suggest that conflicts may be prolonged either to defer the return of HIV-positive troops, or to enable them to gain sufficient money (legally or otherwise) to allow them to purchase anti-retroviral therapies (Elbe 2002, 2003; Heinecken 2003; UNAIDS 2003). A related issue concerned the impact of HIV on peace-keepers, who may be at increased risk from infection (since many of the world's conflicts were in regions with a high prevalence of HIV), and who may also act as vectors for the spread of the disease (UNAIDS 2003: 6).

Finally, concern was expressed that conflict itself may act as a vector for the spread of HIV. Soldiers, already a high-risk group, are willing to engage in even more risky behaviour in conflict regions; incidents of sexual violence increase in conflict; combat injuries may be treated in the field with infected blood; health education and surveillance may be poor in zones of conflict; soldiers returning from conflicts may bring HIV with them; conflicts create migration which may facilitate the spread of HIV; and refugee camps may have poor health education and access to condoms, but are also areas where sexual violence is rife. In addition, HIV may act as a disincentive to end conflicts because of fears that troops from low-prevalence areas may act as a Trojan horse for the spread of the disease on their return (see, e.g., UNAIDS 2003).

The second broad set of reasons why health issues might be a national security problem concerns their ability to affect the internal security of a state. If the domestic economy is damaged, then divisions between rich and poor may be exacerbated. Increased levels of poverty may, in turn, breed social discontent and provide a fertile ground for entrepreneurs of violence. Moreover, confidence in the government, or in the state more generally, may be damaged if public health services are unable to cope. The social contract between a state and its citizens is at risk if the state cannot provide a basic degree of protection; disillusionment and alienation may set in if large numbers start dying and as prospects of survival diminish; absenteeism and high levels of morbidity may rip gaps in the fabric of society. Thus poor health, and in particular epidemic diseases, may pose a security risk to states.

What is again lacking, however, is the empirical evidence to support these arguments. With HIV/AIDS, in particular, a number of states have had very high levels of infection for more than a decade, especially in sub-Saharan Africa. These are also among some of the poorest countries

Box 6.9 Bio-terrorism

The idea of using biological agents (or pathogens) as a weapon to cause disease goes back several hundred years, and was a major concern not least during the Cold War. For much of that period, concern focused upon state use, but in the 1980s and 1990s, a number of political and religious extremist groups used or attempted to use biological weapons. These included a 1984 attempt by followers of Rajneesh Bhagwan to use salmonella to incapacitate voters in Oregon; the 1995 use of sarin in the Tokyo subway by the Aum Shinrikyo cult, which followed their failed attempt at an airborne release of anthrax over Tokyo; letters purporting to contain anthrax spores being sent to abortion clinics and government offices in the US in the late 1990s; and claims that Al Qaeda was attempting to develop an anthrax weapon for mass terror use. At the same time concerns were rising over possible proliferation of biological weapons to states. Intelligence reports suggested that the break-up of the Soviet Union might lead to biological weapons material being sold on the black market to such states as Cuba, Iran, Libya and Syria, while in 1995 a UN Special Commission reported that Iraq had been developing an anthrax weapon during the 1990–1 Gulf War (WHO 2007a: 35–7; Graham 2008: 6–10).

However, the terrorist attacks of 11 September 2001 dramatically increased the sense of risk, demonstrating the willingness and ability of terrorist organizations to inflict mass civilian casualties (see, e.g., Strongin and Redhead 2001). A week later a series of letters were sent to US government officials and media outlets containing anthrax spores, infecting 22 and killing 5. These two events 'showed the potential of bio-terrorism to cause not just death and disability, but social and economic disruption on an enormous scale' (WHO 2007a: 37). The initial focus on anthrax was quickly overtaken by concerns over infectious diseases and especially smallpox, which had been eradicated outside secure laboratory storage in 1979. Unlike non-contagious agents such as anthrax, which require sophisticated methods to infect large numbers of people, smallpox could spread by human-to-human contact; the lag time between infection and symptoms emerging would be several days, meaning rapid exposure of very large numbers of people as those infected wittingly or not continued to move among the population; and its eradication as an endemic disease in 1979 meant that immunization programmes had been stopped, leaving people highly vulnerable to the disease. In a high-profile if somewhat alarmist article, Laurie Garrett wrote 'If the smallpox virus were released today, the majority of the world's population would be defenseless [sic], and given the virus' 30 percent kill rate, nearly two billion people could die . . . The world is thus completely vulnerable to a smallpox attack' (Garrett 2001: 77–8).

Three problems, however, have emerged in responding to the risk of bio-terror. First, there have been clear tensions between an internationally versus a domestically focused strategy. Following the anthrax attacks, the US stepped up its stockpiling of the smallpox vaccine, soon joined by other countries, including the UK. Given the large-scale purchasing by a few states of the vaccine, supplies worldwide were soon in short supply. Similarly, worldwide supplies of the antibiotic Cipro, used to treat anthrax, rapidly became in short supply. This national strategy of stockpiling vaccines raised international concerns over

Continued

hoarding by a few states to the detriment of others. Tensions also arose over the US government's decision to pull out of negotiations on the Biological Weapons Convention (BWC). The priority of the US appeared to be to focus on domestically based security measures, while others argued that a more international approach would yield better results.

This tension is also revealed in the second problem – whether it is better to try and prevent such attacks from happening or whether the priority should be on defence. The former suggests that attention should be given to international cooperation on intelligence and to the use of diplomatic efforts (including arms control) to make the supply and production of such weapons more difficult. In this, public health would be important in monitoring and surveillance of activities, but not the key element in an international strategy. The alternative approach, however, accepts that attacks are likely to be attempted and that a much more nationally focused strategy would be more appropriate. This would use domestic counter-terrorist agencies and 'at-the-border controls' to prevent biological weapons from entering the country, but would also make much greater use of public health systems in defending against such attacks.

The third problem is whether the risk has been overstated. Despite the comparatively recent use of such weapons in Iraq, Japan and the United States, there remain doubts both over how easy it is for sub-state groups to gain access to, or produce, effective weapons and over how easy it is to use them in a manner which might cause significant loss of life. In 2008, the Graham Commission in the US reported that, although the bio-terrorist threat was of concern, 'Because of the difficulty of weaponizing [sic] and disseminating significant quantities of a biological agent in aerosol form, government officials and outside experts believe that no terrorist group currently has an operational capability to carry out a mass-casualty attack. But they could develop that capability quickly . . . [But] given the high level of know-how needed to use disease as a weapon to cause mass casualties, the United States should be less concerned that terrorists will become biologists and far more concerned that biologists will become terrorists' (Graham 2008: 11).

on the planet. Yet there is little evidence to date that high HIV/AIDS prevalence has created destabilizing pressures threatening the security of the state. Nor is the causal link between disease and state insecurity necessarily apparent. Indeed, Barnett and Whiteside (2000) have argued that high prevalence of disease (in their example HIV/AIDS) is not, in and of itself, sufficient to create risks to state security. They argue that it is only if such states also have *both* low social cohesion *and* high levels of poverty/unequal distribution of wealth that they may be at high risk of instability.

The third set of reasons concerns high morbidity and mortality rates. When the number of people at risk reaches exceptional levels, then this moves into the realm of national security, not least because the effective operation of the state may be at risk. The level at which an event becomes sufficiently extraordinary to be considered a security issue, however, is not definable for example as a percentage of the population; rather it is determined inter-subjectively on a case-by-case basis (see Buzan et al. 1997 on the inter-subjective nature of security). But a key feature, for the purposes of this section, is that the cause is portrayed as exogenous to the state; in other words, that it comes from the outside and can therefore be represented as an external threat. Three health issues seem both to meet this necessary condition of externality and to breach the threshold of being outside the ordinary: the spread of existing diseases such as Ebola or West Nile virus to new geographies; the emergence of new, potentially pandemic, diseases such as SARS or a version of H5N1 influenza virus that is readily transmissible human-to-human; and bio-terrorism. Of these, probably only the second has the potential to kill very large numbers of people within a state. But it is not only the level of morbidity that matters, but the sense of risk felt within high-income countries. Thus in the 1990s, when the Ebola virus first appeared in the US, the level of concern and attention far outran what might have been assumed from the number of people realistically at risk from the disease. Similarly, concerns over bio-terrorism may be overstated with doubts over how easy it is for sub-state groups to gain access to, or produce, effective weapons; and over how easy it is to use them in a manner which might cause significant loss of life. But this does not mean that the threat is not *considered* to be very real and of high political salience, resulting in substantial resources being allocated to allay those fears.

In terms of impact, therefore, one can distinguish between the perception of an issue as a health threat and its likely impact upon the state. With both the spread of existing diseases and bio-terrorism, it is clear that people may be at risk; but it is unlikely that these numbers would match those of a major epidemic. What is also crucial to note here is that the concerns are primarily those of Western states, where perhaps the idea of being at risk from disease or from large-scale terrorist atrocities is relatively novel. Much more significant in terms of potential morbidity is the emergence of new diseases with the potential to become pandemics. But, as with the previous section, it is difficult to see how this will necessarily destabilize a state.

Conclusion

This chapter has identified how the traditionally narrow linkage between health and security has been expanded, in both the academic and policy fields, since the late 1990s. It has shown how the links between health and security now encompass a wider range of issues and vulnerabilities than previously. This new development is generally cast in terms of a response to exogenous developments. Crucial to the health security narrative is the argument that new risks have emerged, and have acquired added salience in the context of accelerated globalization. An important element in this narrative is the argument that security's horizons have been broadened beyond the narrow defence of the state against (usually) military threats, to include a more diverse range of risks from novel directions. This has created a space whereby health issues can more easily become a part of the security agenda. That much of the discussion over health and security focuses on a similar range of issues – usually severe and acute epidemic infectious diseases, HIV/AIDS and bio-terrorism – has helped to create the sense that this is a coherent picture where there is agreement over the landscape. What differences do emerge are therefore deemed second order issues concerning how to respond to such risks, rather than the first order scene-setting issues of what is being discussed within the realm of health security in the first place.

As described in chapter 1, the purpose of this book is to ask more critical questions. It starts from the premise that there is nothing 'natural' about the social world, but that it is a construction. From this perspective, narratives which attempt to explain the social world are not objective accounts of observed phenomena, but they help to construct social reality by promoting particular understandings. Crucially, narratives serve a purpose in privileging certain interests and certain ways of seeing the world over others. In this context, the health-security nexus is not a coherent field, but one where there are key differences which are obscured by superficial commonalities. This chapter identifies three distinct ways of seeing the health–security nexus, each of which is different in what it privileges. Thus, *global health security* is concerned with health promotion on a global scale. It is motivated by a belief that risks to public health have been globalized, requiring a response beyond that which individual states are capable of. Its focus is on the emergence of global threats to public health and security, and its primary goal is therefore the well-being of individuals and populations in the face of these threats. *Human security* appears similar in that it is concerned with individuals and communities. Its focus, however, is not on health, but on freedom from fear and from want. Health is thus only a part of the human security agenda, not the focus of it, and other issues may be prioritized, especially poverty alleviation. Therefore, whereas global health security is primarily (and even solely) concerned with the promotion of individual and population health in the face of global risks, human security is concerned with alleviating an individual's or population's fear. Both privilege individuals and populations, but they differ over what they are protecting them from. Finally, *national security* offers a very different perspective on the health–security nexus. Health issues tend to figure on the national security agenda if they are seen as a potential threat to the internal security of the state, have an impact on international stability, or cause exceptional levels of morbidity and/or mortality. What this suggests is that, despite the evolution of the national security perspective, as detailed in this chapter, when it comes to the health–security nexus, the perspective remains heavily state-centric with the interests of the state (and indeed certain powerful states) privileged over those of individuals or communities within the state. What is notably important is how the national security agenda on health has been constructed with limited empirical evidence to support it, suggesting the ability of narratives to construct social realities based on discourse and inter-subjective understandings. The fact that there has been no health crisis leading to state failure has not prevented health issues appearing on certain national security agendas.

Conclusion

Since the 1990s, health and International Relations have been edging closer together within both the academic and policy worlds. After a long history of being largely segregated, the two fields have discovered much common ground and mutual interest. This book has critically examined this developing relationship, located within the rapidly growing but loosely defined subject of 'global health', including their perceived spheres of overlap and what to do about them. Almost all accounts to date have taken the relationship as arising from a necessary response to 'real world' events, centring on the contemporary acceleration of globalization. It has been widely argued, including by one of the current authors (Lee 2000, 2003), that changes to the material world 'out there' are demanding new ways of understanding and responding to that world. Thus, accounts have abounded of globalization creating conditions for emerging and re-emerging diseases spreading more widely and rapidly across the world. Collective responses to this spectre have been sought by bringing together the technical expertise of public health with the political resources of the International Relations community.

While far from denying that globalization is changing the world, and that this changed world is having profound effects on human health, we have argued in this book that this is only part of the story. To tell the fuller story requires us to step away from rationalist accounts of global health and to take a more reflectivist position. For us, the relationship between global health and International Relations is not a 'given'; that is, solely a natural response to evolving circumstances. Rather, we begin by problematizing the relationship itself as something that has been constructed in a particular way, resulting in an emphasis on certain issues and neglect of others, on the prioritizing of some interests over others, on the scientific legitimizing of particular forms of knowledge and methods over others, and on the empowering of specific institutional arrangements over others.

This, in turn, leads to a very different set of questions than has dominated global health debates to date: What are the health needs requiring most urgent attention in a globalizing world? What are the 'best' tools or policies to tackle these global health needs? And how can we (re)build the most effective and efficient institutions to achieve collective action for global health? These are all very important questions but, prior to answering them, a deeper and more critical set of 'why' questions require addressing. Why are certain global health issues deemed as privileged over others (e.g., see chapters 2 and 4)? Why are some tools or policies perceived as preferred over others (e.g., see chapters 3 and 6)? And why are certain institutional arrangements given legitimacy and authority over others (e.g., see chapter 5)?

Seeking to address such 'why' questions as a starting point, we have argued in this book that a range of normatively based frameworks can be observed in global health policy. These frameworks comprise sets of values which shape the articulation of certain ideas, interests and institutions. Moreover, such frameworks even lead to different definitions of global health based on these sets of values. We have described the dominant frames in global health to date (namely security, economism and biomedicine) and how they have been aligned with particular interests within the emerging global political economy. We have argued that these dominant frames have often led to an emphasis by global health actors on acute and severe infectious disease outbreaks over, for example, the impacts of globalization on mental health, accidents and injuries, and a range of non-communicable diseases. The stockpiling of anti-virals and pre-ordering of vaccines, for priority use by selected populations in high-income countries during an influenza pandemic, rather than policies to tackle the socioeconomic conditions that can give rise to zoonosis, can also be understood in terms of these dominant frames providing the ideational basis whereby the global 'haves' can be prioritized over the 'have nots' – most starkly, and rightly or wrongly, the governments of high-income countries have looked first to protecting their own domestic populations over those of other countries (an early example of our position is McInnes and Lee 2006). Yet, it is also apparent that many constituencies, given more or less consideration by the dominant frames in global health policy, do not conform to state boundaries. The poor, regardless of living in a low-, middle- or high-income country, can experience hardship gaining access to health care and essential medicines. It is reported that 46 million Americans lacked health insurance in 2008, and that 275,000 adult deaths would occur between 2010 and 2020 as a result (Andrews 2010). Ring and Brown describe 'the unacceptably large differences between the health of indigenous and non-indigenous populations in developed nations' (Ring and Brown 2003: 404), while Brown (2002) describes the appalling health and safety records of special economic zones the world over geared towards free trade and export processing. Among the beneficiaries of global health policies framed through security, economic or biomedical lenses are transnational providers of health care services and financing, producers of health care goods and services, and the relatively wealthy across all countries able to access them. Overall, the *World Health Report 2008* showed that public spending on health services most often benefits the rich more than the poor in high- and low-income countries alike.

This is not to say that the humanitarian impulse is absent in the policies of governments and other global health actors amid these dominant frames. The significant rise in charitable giving by individuals and philanthropies for global health led by the Bill and Melinda Gates Foundation; the rise of health on the G8, OECD and World Economic Forum agendas; the decision by the UK government to maintain its overseas development aid at existing levels despite widespread cuts in public expenditure in 2010; and, not least, the remarkable flow of students into global health training and education programmes (Brown 2008), all attest to the sincere desire to 'make a difference' to the health of people worldwide. Humanitarian impulses, however, are not exempt from the influence of normative frameworks and, as such, must be equally subject to the 'why' questions described above. The framing of global health in terms of human rights or the social determinants of health, therefore, also reflect particular ways of seeing the world and thus a focus on certain ideas, interests and institutions.

This book has argued for making such normative frameworks explicit as a starting point for fuller debate in global health. Claims based on the primacy of scientific or economic rationalism, on an evidence base limited to certain 'gold standard' methodologies, or other forms of knowledge deemed to be 'common sense' or 'received wisdom', need to be more fully interrogated. Instead, global health can be seen as an arena of competing and contested normative frameworks which are being shaped by, as well as shaping, the 'real world'.

In this spirit, this book has itself been normative in its orientation. It has been critical of the manner in which the relationship between global health and International Relations has been narrowly constructed to date, and of the lack of emphasis on health needs as an overarching governing principle. Our concerns extend to the growing brigade of International Relations scholars who find themselves attracted to the 'plague and pestilence' aspects of global health, as well as members of the public health community seeking to obtain and apply new 'tools' from International Relations. We are, however, encouraged by a number of recent trends which suggest a new relationship might be possible. There are indications that the agenda may be broadening. In September 2011, the UN High-level Meeting on Noncommunicable Diseases was held to give unprecedented attention to health conditions such as cancer, hypertension and diabetes, all of which threaten to dwarf the morbidity and mortality worldwide (63 per cent of total deaths in 2008) caused by infectious diseases. The hopeful may see this as recognition at last of the real burden of disease afflicting a globalizing world, and the start of an overdue shift in research and policy attention. Others have been more cautious, citing the lack of targets, funds and action in the resultant declaration, the impact of the global economic crisis on available resources, the need to apply complex policy interventions to address NCDs and, perhaps most importantly, the strong presence of corporate interests as weighing against such a shift (Cohen 2011). To this daunting mix, we would also add the need to better understand how NCDs and other neglected health conditions have been, and could be, framed to gain political traction. Many NCDs have been typically cast as self-inflicted health problems suffered by individuals who eat, drink or smoke too much. Personal responsibility, rather than stronger regulation or innovative public health initiatives, were deemed lacking. The framing by the World Economic Forum and Harvard School of Public Health (2011) of NCDs as an economic issue, forecast to cost US$47 trillion or 4 per cent of gross domestic product (GDP) over the next twenty years, puts the challenge in a different light. NCDs do not only inflict individuals; they are a collective burden on individual societies and, by extension, the global economy. This economic framing of NCDs would, in turn, suggest that particular policy actions (e.g., pricing, subsidies, taxation) be targeted at certain populations (e.g., young people, adults) to create financial incentives to pursue healthier lifestyles. Alternatively, a social determinants of health approach to NCDs might lead to an emphasis on altering the built environment, to encourage more physical activity, or to review transport, education or agricultural policy.

As well as a broadening agenda, there are signs that dominant normative frameworks may be being challenged. Ongoing efforts to address other global health issues, such as pandemic influenza, health worker migration and access to medicines, can also be more fully understood in the context of competing normative frameworks. The Pandemic Influenza Preparedness Framework (PIPF) agreed in 2011 goes beyond the security risks to high-income countries from a major pandemic, the biomedical need to secure virus samples to develop appropriate vaccines, and the need to provide pharmaceutical manufacturers sufficient economic incentives to invest in production facilities, to recognizing the core problem of inequitable access to such vaccines. In addition to a commitment to create stockpiles of anti-viral drugs and vaccines for use by countries most affected in an influenza pandemic, the PIPF urges member states to address the inherent structural problems inhibiting expansion of capacity in the vaccine manufacturing industry. The adoption of the WHO Global Code of Practice on the International Recruitment of Health Personnel in 2010 offers another framework for addressing a major social justice issue in global health. As Emily deRiel of the nongovernmental organization Health Alliance International writes,

> It doesn't seem fair that wealthy countries – which have the most health workers per capita, the lowest disease burden and can better afford to train more health workers of their own – should take health workers from poor countries that desperately need them. (deRiel 2010)

At the same time, the organization recognizes that 'who can begrudge health workers the opportunity to take a job abroad that offers better pay, better working conditions, and a chance to develop their careers and support their families. The right to migrate is a human right.' Both issues illustrate that multiple and competing frameworks come into play, change can occur over time regarding the prevailing dominant normative framework, and that negotiating institutional arrangements for global health governance is a process of reconciling and even combining such frameworks.

Another apparent trend in global health is the emergent and deterritorialized nature of its polity. What constituencies make up global health? As described above, the traditional distinction between 'developed' and 'developing' countries increasingly fails to capture the distribution of health costs and benefits in a globalizing world. The so-called emerging economies, along with other middle-income countries, are predicted to be increasingly influential players in global health, with their own needs, agendas and perspectives. Interest has, for example, begun to focus on the role of the BRIC states (Brazil, Russia, India and China) as emerging powers in global health governance (Lee et al. 2010; Ng and Ruger 2010), and on whether the G20, with its greater plurality, may supersede the G8. In this respect, the Oslo Declaration is an example of new coalitions of states forming within global health.

Moreover, if globalization is deterritorialization (see chapter 1), this requires us to redefine the boundaries of its constituencies and their corresponding health needs in new ways. Individuals may have multiple identities that cut across national, ethnic, gender, religious and other lines. Thus, a young female worker employed in a non-unionized factory located in a special economic zone in India experiences a mixture of costs and benefits to her health. She may be exposed to unsafe working conditions, have to travel and live in risky social settings, and have limited access to nutritious food or clean water. However, she may also have the opportunity to earn increased income, and have improved access to health education and services from the employment site.

Social groups also reflect the multiplicity of identity and health needs in global health. Civil society organizations, patient groups, trade unions, religious organizations, industry associations, academic institutions, professional bodies and many other groups inhabit the global health polity. It has been observed that this emerging global health civil society has the opportunity to express their views through major gatherings such as the International Aids Conference, World Conference on Tobacco or Health, and the Global Forum for Health Research. In 2010, the annual UN Conference with civil society groups focused on global health.[1] As discussed in chapter 5, there remains much debate about the genuine capacity of such actors to have a voice in global health policy making, and the need to democratize key institutions such as the WHO. We recognize too that civil society is not necessarily always a progressive force, and that greater plurality can mean an even greater lack of coherence in global health action. We argue that the capacity to acknowledge, and where possible reconcile, the multiple normative frameworks represented by this plurality, will need to be an essential feature of global health governance in future as the boundaries dividing the 'haves' and 'have nots' become more nuanced.

Finally, we observe an encouraging trend towards the application of social constructivist approaches to more deeply interrogate the nature of global health, as an emerging academic field and subject of committed action. We need to keep asking the 'why' questions, not as a mischievous child might do, but as scholars, policy makers and practitioners committed to improving the health of populations worldwide.

Notes

Chapter 1

1. For general references for this chapter, see Surel (2000), Fauci (2007) and Janes and Corbett (2011).
2. See http://www.theglobalfund.org/en/.
3. See http://www.ghi.gov/.
4. This includes films such as *Outbreak* (1995) and *Contagion* (2011).
5. For example, in its assessment of the future 'strategic and operational context' for the US military, the only health issue that the US Joint Forces Command report cites is pandemic diseases (USJFC 2010).
6. We recommend, for example, Robertson (1992), Held et al. (1999) and Baylis and Smith (1997).
7. See http://www.globalizationandhealth.com/about.
8. From http://www.csih.org/en/aboutus/index.asp.

Chapter 2

1. This book distinguishes between international relations as a practice and International Relations as an academic discipline, though on occasion the two are not distinct and their use may be fungible.
2. For general references, see Gordenker (1995), Price-Smith (2002), Dietrich (2007) and WHO (2011).
3. For example, risks can arise through the destruction of hospitals affecting the provision of secondary health care; through refugee flows establishing new risks as vectors for the spread of disease; and through the difficulties in supplying drugs in conflict zones affecting primary health care.
4. Notable exceptions are Jacobson (1974) and Siddiqi (1995).
5. For a review of this literature, see Lee (2010).
6. There is no adequate definition of 'the West', nor of 'North–South'. Common usage is generally vague, with the 'West' generally referring to 'advanced' liberal democracies and/or high income states in Europe, North America and perhaps Japan and Australasia. While 'North–South' has lost some of its original value as a geographical analogue to 'rich/poor', it still tends to be used in that sense with middle income countries such as Brazil and India sitting rather uncomfortably between the two poles. Given that much of the literature and policies we are inter-

ested in maintain this vague usage, we have followed suit since attempting a single definition would not have helped in our analysis.

7. An acute health condition refers to the timeframe of its onset and duration. An acute condition lasts for a relatively short period of time, but can begin rapidly and have intense symptoms. This contrasts with chronic conditions, which have a longer timeframe of onset and duration, and generally less intense symptoms.

8. A severe health condition is one that causes a serious, and even life-threatening, impact on the sufferer. Diseases can be described as mild or severe depending on the seriousness of their impact on an individual's capacity to function.

9. These include the Centre on International Relations and Health, Aberystwyth University; Global Health and Foreign Policy Initiative, Nitze School of Advanced International Studies, Johns Hopkins University; Global Health and Security Programme, Stockholm International Peace Research Institute; and the Centre on Global Health Security, Chatham House.

10. It is interesting to note that the global health agenda is not aligned with this narrow focus, although donors have heavily focused on these infectious disease threats plus HIV/AIDS. It is a good example of how ideas influence practice.

11. WHO, updated June 2011. http://www.who.int/mediacentre/factsheets/fs310/en/index.html. WHO explains the omission of tobacco from this list: 'Tobacco use is a major cause of many of the world's top killer diseases – including cardiovascular disease, chronic obstructive lung disease and lung cancer. In total, tobacco use is responsible for the death of almost one in 10 adults worldwide. Smoking is often the hidden cause of the disease recorded as responsible for death.'

12. A variety of slightly different versions of 'ABC' were developed over a number of years by different bodies, but the simplest was 'abstain, be faithful, use a condom'.

13. See http://hivpreventiontoolkit.unaids.org/Knowledge_Epidemic.aspx.

14. This can also lead to geographies of perception of risk. This leads to a belief that one can somehow barricade state borders to keep out disease, much like plague victims were bricked up behind walls. Or that screening of population movements can be an effective strategy. The naming of the US security agency as the US Department of Homeland Security, which covers health threats from abroad, reinforces this perceived geography. This geography ignores the global structural factors that are broader determinants of these health threats. Policies based on such perceptions are also ineffective in an interconnected world.

15. See http://www.world-heart-federation.org/cardiovascular-health/cardio vascular-disease-risk-factors/.

16. According to the WHO: 'The right to health means that governments must generate conditions in which everyone can be as healthy as

possible. Such conditions range from ensuring availability of health services, healthy and safe working conditions, adequate housing and nutritious food. The right to health does not mean the right to be healthy.' See WHO (2007e).

17. In addition there have been expressions of scepticism over whether the link was 'real' and/or how important it might be. This view has come especially from the foreign and security policy community, but has rarely been expressed in printed form.

Chapter 4

1. Cited in Plunkett's Health Care Industry, Market research, business trends and statistics analysis, and business development support. http://plunkettresearch.com/health%20care%20medical%20market%20research/industry%20and%20business%20data.
2. See http://www.contractpharma.com/contents/view/33747.

Chapter 5

1. See http://www.ghsi.ca/english/background.asp.
2. Jamison et al. (eds.) (1993) is described on The Gates Notes (the official website of Bill Gates), available at http://www.thegatesnotes.com/Books/Health/Disease-Control-Priorities-in-Developing-Countries.
3. See http://www.grandchallenges.org.ABOUT/Pages/Overview.aspx.
4. Cochrane Collection, see http://www.cochrane.org/about-us.
5. See https://apps.who.int/director-general/biographies/murray_chris.html
6. See http://www.who.int/healthmetrics/about/governance/en/index.html
7. See http://www.ghwatch.org/who-watch/ghg
8. See http://www.phmovement.org/sites/www.phmovement.org/files/PHMLetter2WHADelegates110516.pdf.
9. The Kaiser Family Foundation, a leader in health policy analysis, health journalism and communication, is dedicated to filling the need for trusted, independent information on the biggest health issues facing our nation and its people. The Foundation is a non-profit private operating foundation, based in Menlo Park, California.

Chapter 6

1. See also UNDP (1994), particularly 22–24.
2. For more on this see the section on development in chapter 3.
3. See, for example, figures on US casualties in major wars at http://www.pbs.org/greatwar/resources/casdeath_pop.html and also Cirillo (2008).

Conclusion

1. See http://www.un.org/apps/news/story.asp?NewsID=33784&Cr=akasaka&Cr1=

References

Aginam, Obijiofor (2010) 'Global health governance, intellectual property and access to essential medicines: opportunities and impediments for South-South cooperation', *Global Health Governance*, 4(1). Available at: http://www.ghgj.org.

Akin, John S. and Nancy Birdsall and David M. De Ferranti (1987) *Financing Health Services in Developing Countries: An Agenda for Reform*. Washington, DC: World Bank.

Anderson, Matthew R., Lanny Smith and Victor W. Sidel (2005) 'What is Social Medicine', *Monthly Review*, 56(8). Available at: http://www. monthlyreview.org/0105anderson.htm.

Ando, Gus (2011) 'Global Healthcare and Pharma in 2012: Ten predictions for the year ahead', IHS. Available at: http://healthcare.blogs.ihs.com/ 2011/12/20/global-healthcare-and-pharma-in-2012-ten-predictions-for-the-year-ahead/.

Andresen, Steinar (2002) *Leadership Change in the World Health Organization: Potential for Increased Effectiveness?* Fridtjof Nansens Institutt, Norway. Available at: www.fni.no/doc&pdf/FNI-R0802.pdf.

Andrews, Michelle (2010) 'Deaths rising for lack of insurance, study finds', *New York Times*, 26 February. Available at: http://prescriptions.blogs. nytimes.com/2010/02/26/deaths-rising-due-to-lack-of-insurance-study-finds/.

Anon (2011) 'Let's be straight up about the alcohol industry', *PLoS Medicine*, 8(5). Available at: http://www.plosmedicine.org/article/info:doi/10.1371/ journal.pmed.1001041.

Anon (no date) 'Donor and mutual accountability in scaling up for better health', Report to the High-Level Forum on the Health MDGs. Available at: http://www.hlfhealthmdgs.org/Documents/070605IsenmannMutualA ccountabilityFINAL.pdf.

Anyangwe, Stella C.E. and Chipayeni Mtonga (2007) 'Inequities in the global health workforce: the greatest impediment to health in sub-Saharan Africa', *International Journal of Environmental Research and Public Health*, 4(2), 93–100.

Armitage, Richard L. and Joseph S. Nye (2007) *CSIS Commission on Smart Power, A Smarter more Secure America*, Washington, DC: Center for Strategic and

International Studies. Available at: http://www.csis.org/files/media/csis/pubs/071106_csissmartpowerreport.pdf.

ASCI [AIDS, Security and Conflict Initiative] (2009) *HIV/AIDS, Security and Conflict: New Realities, New Responses*, ASCI Final Report. Available at: http://asci.researchhub.ssrc.org/rdb/asci-hub.

Ashton, J. R. (2006) 'Virchow misquoted, part-quoted, and the real McCoy', *Journal of Epidemiology and Community Health*, 60, 671.

Axworthy, Lloyd (1997) 'Canada and human security: the need for leadership', *International Journal*, 52(2), 183–96.

Axworthy, Lloyd (2001) 'Human security and global governance: putting people first', *Global Governance*, 7(1), 19–24.

Azad, Ghulam Nabi (2011) 'BRIC nations pledge cheaper drugs for developing nations', *The Times of India*, 12 July.

Baker, Major Jay B. (2007) 'Medical diplomacy in full-spectrum operations', *Military Review*, 26, 67–73.

Baker, Michael G. and Andrew M. Forsyth (2007) 'The new International Health Regulations: a revolutionary change in global health security', *New Zealand Medical Journal*, 120 (1267). Available at: http://www.nzma.org.nz/jurnal/120-1267/2872.

Balzacq, Thierry (2005) 'The three faces of securitization: political agency, audience and context', *European Journal of International Relations*, 11(2), 171–201.

Barbour, Virginia, Paul Chinnock, Barbara Cohen and Gavin Yamey (2006) 'The impact of open access upon public health', *Bulletin of the World Health Organization*, 84(5), 339–40.

Barnett, Tony and Alan Whiteside (2000) 'The Jaipur Paradigm: a conceptual framework for understanding social susceptibility and vulnerability to HIV', *South African Medical Journal*, 90, 1098–101.

Basch, Paul F. (1999) *Textbook of International Health*, 2nd edn. Oxford: Oxford University Press.

Bathurst, Ian and Chris Hentschel (2006) 'Medicines for Malaria Venture: sustaining antimalarial drug development', *Trends in Parasitology*, 22(7), 301–7.

Batley, Richard and George Larbi (2004) *The Changing Role of Government, The Reform of Public Services in Developing Countries*. London: Palgrave Macmillan.

Baylis, John and Steve Smith (eds.) (1997) *The Globalization of World Politics, An Introduction to International Relations*. Oxford: Oxford University Press.

Beaglehole Robert and R. Bonita (2010) 'What is global health?', *Global Health Action*, 3, 5142.

Beckett, Andy (2010) 'Inside the Bill and Melina Gates Foundation', *The Guardian*, 12 July.

Béhague, Dominique B., Charlotte Tawiah, Mikey Rosato, Télésphore Some and Joanna Morrison (2009) 'Evidence-based policy-making: The implications of globally-applicable research for context-specific problem-solving in developing countries', *Social Science and Medicine*, 69(10), 1539–45.

Bell, Ruth, Sebastian Taylor and Michael Marmot (2010) 'Global health governance: Commission on social determinants of health and the imperative for change', *Journal of Law, Medicine and Ethics*, 38(3), 470–85.

Bernstein, Michael and Myra Sessions (2007) *A Trickle or a Flood: Commitments and Disbursements for HIV/AIDS from the global Fund, PEPFAR and the World Bank's Multi-Country AIDS Program (MAP)*. Washington DC: Center for Global Development.

Biritwum, R.B. (1994) 'The cost of sustaining the Ghana's "cash and carry" system of health care financing at a rural health center', *West African Journal of Medicine*, 13, 124–7.

Bisaillon, Laura M. (2010) 'Human rights consequences of mandatory HIV screening policy of newcomers to Canada', *Health and Human Rights*, 12(2), 119–34.

Blas, Eric and M.E. Limbambala (2001) 'User-payment, decentralization and health service utilization in Zambia', *Health Policy and Planning*, 16(Suppl 2), 19–28.

Bloom, Barry R., Catherine M. Michaud, John R. La Montagne and Lone Simonsen (2006) 'Priorities for global research and development of interventions' in D.T. Jamison, J.G. Breman, A.R. Measham et al. (eds.) *Disease Control Priorities in Developing Countries*, 2nd edn. Washington, DC: World Bank.

Bonventre, Eugene V., Kathleen H. Hicks and Stacy M. Okutani (2009) *US National Security and Global Health: An Analysis of Global Health Engagement by the US Department of Defense*. Washington, DC: Center for Strategic and International Studies.

Brewer, Timothy (no date) 'What's in a name?'. Available at: http://www.mcgill.ca/globalhealth/director-message.

Brock Tina, David Taylor and Tana Wuliji (2007) *Curbing the Tobacco Pandemic: The Global Role for Pharmacy*. London: School of Pharmacy, University of London and International Pharmaceutical Federation.

Brower, Jennifer and Peter Chalk (2003) *The Global Threat of New and Re-emerging Infectious Diseases: Reconciling US National Security and Public Health*. Santa Monica, CA: RAND Corporation.

Brown, David (2008) 'For a global generation, public health is a hot field', *Washington Post*, 19 September. Available at: http://www.washingtonpost.com/wp-dyn/content/article/2008/09/18/AR2008091804145.html.

Brown, Garrett D. (2002) 'The global threats to workers' health and safety on the job', *Social Justice*, 29 (3), 12–25. Available at: http://mhssn.igc.org/gbrown.htm.

Brown, Theodore M., Marcos Cueto and Elizabeth Fee (2006) 'The World Health Organization and the transition from international to global public health', *American Journal of Public Health*, 96(1), 62–72.

Brownell, Kelly D. and Kenneth E. Warner (2009) 'The perils of ignoring history: Big tobacco played dirty and millions died. How similar is big food?', *Milbank Quarterly*, 87(1), 259–94.

Brundtland, Gro Harlem (1999) 'Why investing in health is good politics', speech to the Council on Foreign Relations, New York, 6 December. Available at: http://www.who.int/director-general/speeches/1999/english/19991206_new_york.html.

Brundtland, Gro Harlem (2002) 'AIDS and global security', speech to the Nobel Centenary Roundtable, 25 January. Available at: http://www.who.iny/director-general/speeches/2002/english/20020125_nobelroundtable.html.

Brundtland, Gro Harlem (2003) 'Global health and international security', *Global Governance*, 9(4), 417–23.

Buckup, Sebastian (2008) 'Global public-private partnerships against neglected diseases: building governance structures for effective outcomes', *Health Economics, Policy and Law*, 3(1), 31–50.

Bull, Benedicte and Desmond McNeill (2007) 'Global partnerships for health: health for all or more "Big Pharma"?' In B. Bull and D. McNeill (eds.) *Development Issues in Global Governance, Public-Private Partnerships and Market Multilateralism.* New York: Routledge.

Bull, Hedley (1977) *The Anarchical Society: A Study of Order in World Politics.* London: Macmillan.

Burns, Andrew, Dominique van der Mensbrugghe and Hans Timmer (2008) *Evaluating the Economic Consequences of Avian Influenza.* Available at: http://siteresources.worldbank.org/EXTAVIANFLU/Resources/EvaluatingAHIeconomics_2008.pdf.

Busby, Joshua W. (2007), 'Bono made Jesse Helms cry: Jubilee2000, debt relief and moral action in international politics', *International Studies Quarterly*, 51(2), 247–75.

Buse, Kent (1994), 'The World Bank', *Health Policy and Planning*, 9(1), 95–9.

Buse, Kent and Andrew M. Harmer (2007) 'Seven habits of highly effective global public-private health partnerships: Practice and potential', *Social Science and Medicine*, 64, 259–71.

Buse, Kent and Gill Walt (2000) 'Global public-private partnerships: Part 1 – A new development in health?', *Bulletin of the World Health Organization*, 78(4), 549–61.

Busfield, Joan (2005) 'The globalization of the pharmaceutical industry'. In Kelley Lee and Jeff Collin (eds.) *Global Change and Health.* Maidenhead: Open University Press, 95–110.

Bush, George W. (2003) 'President speaks on fighting global and domestic HIV/AIDS'. Available at: http://www.state.gov.

Buzan, Barry (1991) *People, States and Fear*, 2nd edn. Hemel Hempstead: Harvester Wheatsheaf.

Buzan, Barry, Ole Waever and Jap de Wilde (1997) *Security: A New Framework for Analysis.* Boulder, CO: Lynne Rienner.

Cabinet Office [UK] (2008) *The National Security Strategy of the United Kingdom: Security in an Interdependent World.* Available at: http://interactive.cabinetoffice.gov.uk/documents/security/national_security_strategy.pdf.

Cabinet Office [UK] (2010) *A Strong Britain in an Age of Uncertainty: The National Security Strategy*. Available at: http://www.cabinetoffice.gov.uk/sites/default/files/resources/national-security-strategy.pdf.

Carlson, Cindy (2004) 'Mapping Global Health Partnerships', *Global Health Programme Study Paper No. 1*, London: DfID Health Resource Centre. Available at: http://www2.ohchr.org/english/issues/development/docs/WHO_1.pdf.

Cerny, Phil G. (1996) 'What next for the state?'. In E. Kofman and G. Youngs (eds.) *Globalization Theory and Practice*. London: Pinter, 123–37.

Chalker, Baroness Linda (1996) 'ODA: new aims and priorities', unpublished speech at Royal Institute of International Affairs, Chatham House, London, 14 February.

Chan, Lai-Han, Lucy Chen, Jin Xu (2010) 'China's engagement with global health diplomacy: was SARS a watershed?', *PLoS Medicine*, 7 (4). Available at: http://www.plosmedicine.org/article/info%3Adoi%2F10.1371%2Fjournal.pmed.1000266.

Chan, Margaret (2011) 'Aid is still not as effective as it ought to be', opening remarks of WHO Director-General at a consultation on global health governance, Geneva, 11 March.

Chang, Alfred E., Patricia A. Ganz, Daniel F. Hayes, Timothy Kinsella, Harvey I. Pass, Joan H. Schiller, Richard M. Stone and Victor Strecher (eds.) (2005) *Oncology: An Evidence-based Approach*. New York: Springer.

Chen, Lincoln C. (2004) 'Health as a human security priority for the 21st century', paper for Helsinki Process Human Security Track III. Available at: http://www.helsinkiprocess.fi/netcomm/ImgLib/24/89/LCHelsinkiPaper12%5b1%5d.6.04.pdf.

Chen, Lincoln C., Jennifer Leaning and Vasant Narashimhan (eds.) (2003) *Global Health Challenges for Human Security*. Cambridge, MA: Harvard University Press.

China Research and Development (2011) *Research Report on China's and Global Blood Products Industry, 2011–2012*. Available at: http://www.shcri.com/upImgFile/20101221636181010152-Research%20Report%20on%20Global%20and%20Chinas%20Blood%20Products%20Industry%202011-2012.pdf.

CIA [Central Intelligence Agency] (2000) *The Global Infectious Disease Threat and Its Implications for the United States*, National Intelligence Estimate NIE99-17D. Available at: http://www.cia.gov/cia/publications/nie/report/nie99-17d.html.

Cirillo, Vincent J. (2008) 'Two faces of death: fatalities from disease and combat in America's principal wars, 1775 to present', *Perspectives in Biology and Medicine*, 51(1), 121–33.

Clinton, Hillary (2010) *The Global Health Initiative: the next phase of American leadership in health around the world*, speech to the School of Advanced Studies, Johns Hopkins University, Washington, DC, 16 August. Available at: http://www.state.gov/secretary/rm/2010/08/146002.htm.

Cockerham, William and Geoffrey Cockerham (2010) *Health and Globalization*. London: Polity.

Cohen, Deborah (2011) 'Will industry derail the UN summit?', *British Medical Journal*, 343, 23 August.

Cohen, Jon (2006) 'Policy network for HIV/AIDS, Tanzania', *Science*, 13 January. Available at: http://www.sciencemag.org/cgi/reprint/311/5758/162.pdf

Coker, Richard (2003) *Migration, Public Health and Compulsory Screening for TB and HIV*. London: IPPR.

Colgan, Ann-Louise (2002) 'Hazardous to health: The World Bank and IMF in Africa', Africa Action Position Paper. Available at: http://africaaction.org/action/sap0204.htm.

Collier, Stephen J. and Andrew Lakoff (2008) 'The problem of securing health', in A. Lakoff and S. J. Collier (eds.) *Biosecurity Interventions: Global Health and Security in Question*. New York: Columbia University Press.

Collin, Jeff, Kelley Lee and Karen Bissell (2002) 'The framework convention on tobacco control: the politics of global health governance', *Third World Quarterly*, 23(2), 265–82.

Contract Pharma (2010) 'Top 20 Pharmaceutical Companies Report'. Available at: http://www.contractpharma.com/contents/view/33747.

Cook, Robin (2000) 'Foreign policy and national interest', speech delivered to the Royal Institute of International Affairs, Chatham House, London, 28 January. Available at: http://www/fco.gov.uk.

Cooper, Andrew F., John J. Kirton and Ted Schrecker (eds.) (2009) *Governing Global Health*. Aldershot: Ashgate.

Cox, Robert W. (1981) 'Social forces, states and world order: beyond International Relations theory', *Millennium: Journal of World Politics*, 10(2), 126–55.

Cox, Robert W. (1987) *Production, Power and World Order, Social Forces in the Making of History*. New York: Columbia University Press.

Curley, Melissa and Nicholas Thomas (2004) 'Human security and public health in Southeast Asia: the SARS outbreak', *Australian Journal of International Affairs*, 58(1), 17–32.

Cutler, David and Grant Miller (2005) 'The role of public health improvements in health advances: the twentieth-century United States', *Demography*, 42(1), 1–22.

Davies, Philip (2004) 'Is evidence based government possible?', paper presented at 4th Annual Campbell Collaboration Colloquium, 19 February. Available at: http://www.nationalschool.gov.uk/policyhub/downloads/JerryLeeLecture1202041.pdf

Davies, Sara E. (2010) *Global Politics of Health*. Oxford: Polity.

DeAngeli, Catherine D. and Phil B. Fontanarosa (2010) 'Strengthening the credibility of clinical research', *Lancet*, 376(9737), 234.

Deloitte South East Asia (2011) *Private Healthcare Providers: The Prognosis for Growth*. Available at: http://www.deloitte.com/assets/Dcom-Indonesia/Local%20Assets/Documents/Private_Healthcare_Provider.pdf.

Department of Foreign Affairs and Trade [Australia] (2003) *Advancing the National Interest: Australia's Foreign and Trade White Paper*. Available at: http://www.dfat.gov.au/ani.

Department of Health [UK] (2008a) *Health is Global: A UK Government Strategy 2008–13*. London: HMSO.

Department of Health [UK] (2008b) *Tackling Health Inequalities*. London: HMSO.

Department for International Development [UK] (2000) *Eliminating World Poverty: Making Globalisation Work for the Poor*. London: TSO.

deRiel, Emily (2010) 'Can a code of practice improve the fairness of international recruitment of health care workers?', Health Alliance International, University of Washington. Available at: http://www.healthallianceinternational.org/blog/post/can-a-code-of-practice-improve-the-fairness-of-international-recruitment.

Deudney, David (1990) 'The case against linking environmental degradation and national security', *Millennium: Journal of World Politics*, 19(3), 461–76.

Dhillon, Ibadat S., Margaret Clark and Robert Kapp (2010) *Innovations in Cooperation: A Guidebook on Bilateral Agreements to Address Health Worker Migration*. Aspen, CO: Aspen Institute.

Dietrich, John W. (2007) 'The politics of PEPFAR: The President's Emergency Plan for AIDS Relief', *Ethics and International Affairs*, 21(3), 277–92.

Docteur, Elizabeth and Howard Oxley (2003) 'Health-Care Systems: Lessons from the Reform Experience', OECD Health Working Papers, Paris, No. 9. Available at: http://www.oecd.org/dataoecd/5/53/22364122.pdf

Doughton, Sandi and Kristi Heim (2011) 'Does Gates funding of media taint objectivity?', *Seattle Times*, 19 February. Available at: http://seattletimes.nwsource.com/html/localnews/2014280379_gatesmedia.html.

Downer, Alexander (2003) 'Why health matters in foreign policy'. Available at: http://www.foreignminister.gov.au/speeches/2003.

Doyal, Lesley (1979) *The Political Economy of Health*. London: Pluto Press.

Drager, Nick and David P. Fidler (2007) 'Foreign policy, trade and health: at the cutting edge of global health diplomacy', *Bulletin of the World Health Organization*, 85(3), 162. Available at: http://www.who.int/bulletin/volumes/85/3/07-041079/en/index.html.

Duffield, Mark (2001) *Global Governance and the New Wars*. London: Zed.

ECDC [European Centre for Disease Prevention and Control] (2004) *Mission*, Article Three, Founding Regulation, EC851/2004.

Eisenberg, Pablo (2011) 'As it seeks a new leader, Council on Foundations must take risks', *Chronicle of Philanthropy*, 28 July. Available at: http://philanthropy.com/article/Philanthropy-Needs-a-Leader/128345.

Elbe, Stefan (2002) 'HIV/AIDS and the changing landscape of war in Africa', *International Security*, 27(2), 159–77.

Elbe, Stefan (2003) *The Strategic Implications of HIV/AIDS*, Adelphi Paper 357, Oxford: Oxford University Press for the International Institute for Strategic Studies.

Elbe, Stefan (2006) 'Should HIV/AIDS be securitized? The ethical dilemmas of linking HIV/AIDS and security', *International Studies Quarterly*, 50(1), 119–44.

Elbe, Stefan (2009) *Virus Alert: Security, Governmentality and the AIDS Pandemic.* New York: Columbia University Press.

Elbe, Stefan (2010) *Security and Global Health: Toward the Medicalization of Insecurity.* Cambridge: Polity.

Enemark, Christian P. (2010) 'Law in the time of anthrax: biosecurity lessons from the United States', *Journal of Law and Medicine*, 17(5), 748–60.

Enloe, Cynthia (1989) *Bananas, Beaches and Bases: Making Feminist Sense of International Politics.* London: Pandora.

Epsicom Healthcare Intelligence (2011) *The Outlook for Pharmaceuticals in Brazil, Russia, India and China.* Rockville, MD: MarketResearch.com.

Ernst & Young (2010) *Ernst & Young's 24th Annual Report on the Biotech Industry.* Available at: http://www.ey.com/US/en/Newsroom/News-releases/Biotech-industry-showing-resilience-despite-challenging-conditions.

Evans, Tony (2002) 'A human right to health?', *Third World Quarterly*, 23(2), 197–215.

Fallon, William J. and Helene D. Gayle (2010) *Report of the Commission on Smart Global Health Policy.* Washington, DC: Center for Strategic and International Studies.

Fang, Pengqian, Siping Dong, Jingjing Xiao, Chaojie Liu, Xianwei Feng and Yiping Wang (2010) 'Regional inequality in health and its determinants: evidence from China', *Health Policy*, 94(1), 14–25.

Farmer, Paul E. and Nicole Gastineau Campos (2007) 'New malaise: Bioethics and human rights in the global era', *Journal of Law, Medicine and Ethics*, 32(2), 243–51.

Fauci, Anthony S. (2007) 'The expanding global health agenda: a welcome development', *Nature Medicine*, 13, 1169–71. Available at: http://www.nature.com/nm/journal/v13/n10/full/nm1646.html.

FCO [UK Foreign and Commonwealth Office] (2003) *UK International Priorities: A Strategy for the FCO, Cm 6052.* London: HMSO.

Feinsilver, Julie M. (2009) 'Cuba's medical diplomacy', in M.A. Font (compiler) *A Changing Cuba in a Changing World.* New York: CUNY Bildner Center.

Feldbaum, Harley and Joshua Michaud (2010) 'Health diplomacy and the enduring relevance of foreign policy interests', *PLoS Medicine*, 7(4). Available at: http://www.plosmedicine.org/article/info:doi%2F10.1371%2Fjournal. pmed.1000226

Feldbaum, Harley, Kelley Lee and Joshua Michaud (2010) 'Global health and foreign policy', *Epidemiological Review*, 32(1), 82–92.

Fidler, David P. (2003) 'SARS: Political pathology of the first post-Westphalian plague', *Journal of Law, Medicine and Ethics*, 31(4), 485–505.

Fidler, David P. (2004) 'Caught between paradise and power: Public health, pathogenic threats, and the axis of illness', *McGeorge Law Review*, 35(1), 45–104.

Fidler, David P. (2006a) 'Biosecurity: Friend or foe for public health governance?', in A. Bashford (ed.) *Medicine at the Border: Disease Globalization and Security from 1859 to the Present*. Basingstoke: Palgrave Macmillan.

Fidler, David P. (2006b) 'Health as foreign policy: harnessing globalization for health', *Health Promotion International*, 21(Special Supplement I), 51–8.

Fidler, David P. (2008) 'Influenza virus samples, international law and global health diplomacy', *Emerging Infectious Diseases*, 14(1), 88–94.

Fidler, David P. (2010) 'The challenge of global health governance', working paper, New York: Council on Foreign Relations.

Fidler, David P. (2011) 'Navigating the global health terrain: mapping global health diplomacy', *Asian Journal of WTO and International Health Law and Policy*, 6(1), 1–43. Available at: http://ssrn.com/abstract=1822908.

Fidler, David P. and Nick Drager (2009) 'Global health and foreign policy: Strategic opportunities and challenges', background paper for the Secretary General's Report on Global Health and Foreign Policy. Available at: http://www.who.int/trade/events/UNGA_Background_Rep3_2.pdf.

Fidler, David P. and Lawrence Gostin (2006) 'The new International Health Regulations: an historic development for international law and public health', *Journal of Law, Medicine and Ethics*, 34(1), 85–94.

Fidler, David P. and Lawrence Gostin (2008) *Biosecurity in the Global Age: Biological Weapons, Public Health and the Rule of Law*. Stanford, CA: Stanford University Press.

Flanagan, Robert J. (2006) *Globalization and Labor Conditions: Working Conditions and Worker Rights in a Global Economy*. Oxford: Oxford University Press.

Fleck, Fiona (2003) 'How SARS changed the world in less than six months', *Bulletin of the World Health Organization*, 81(8), 625–6.

Foreman, Christopher H. (1994) *Plagues, Products and Politics: Emergent Public Health Hazards and National Policymaking*. Washington, DC: Brookings Institution.

Franco-Geraldo, Alvaro, Marco Palma and Carlos Alvarez-Dardet (2006) 'The effect of structural adjustment on health conditions in Latin America and the Caribbean, 1980–2000', *Pan American Journal of Public Health*, 19(5), 291–9.

Freedman, Lawrence (1998) 'International security: Changing targets', *Foreign Policy*, 110, 48–63.

Freeman, Charles W. and Xiaoqing Lu Boynton (eds.) (2011) *China's Emerging Global Health and Foreign Aid Engagement in Africa*. Washington DC: Center for Strategic and International Studies.

Frist, Senator William H. (2008) 'Medicine as a currency for peace through global health diplomacy', *Yale Law and Policy Review*, 26(1), 209–29.

G8 [Group of Eight] (2011) *Deauville Accountability Report: G8 Commitments on Health and Food Security: State of Delivery and Results*. Available at: http://www.g8.utoronto.ca/summit/2011deauville/deauville/2011-deauville-accountability-report.pdf

Gagne, Joshua J. (2011) 'Commentary: How many "me too" drugs is too many?' *Journal of the American Medical Association*, 305(7), 711–12.

Garrett, Laurie (1994) *The Coming Plague: Newly Emergent Diseases in a World Out of Balance*. New York: Farrar, Straus and Giroux.

Garrett, Laurie (2001) 'The nightmare of bioterrorism', *Foreign Affairs*, 80(1), 76–89.

Garrett, Laurie (2007) 'The challenge of global health', *Foreign Affairs*, 86(1), 14–38.

Gercheva, Dafina, Joe Hooper and Alexandra Windisch-Graetz (no date) 'Towards more effective state institutions', New York: UN Development Programme. Available at: http://www.developmentandtransition.net/Article.35+M5fe7c14e841.0.html.

GHSI [Global Health Security Initiative] (no date) Available at: http://www.ghsi.ca/english/background.asp.

Gill, Stephen and David Law (1988) *The Global Political Economy, Perspectives, Problems and Policies*. New York: Harvester Wheatsheaf.

Gilpin, Robert (1987) *The Political Economy of International Relations*. Princeton, NJ: Princeton University Press.

Gleneagles Communiqué (2005) *The Gleneagles Communiqué 2005*. Available at: http://www.unglobalcompact.org/docs/about_the_gc/government_support/PostG8_Gleneagles_Communique.pdf.

Global Forum for Health Research (2004) *10/90 Gap Report 2003–2004*, Geneva.

Global Health Council (no date) 'What we do', Available at: http://www.globalhealth.org/view_top.php3?id=234.

Global Industry Analysts Inc. (2010) *Blood Banking and Blood Products, A Global Business Strategic Report*. Available at: http://www.strategyr.com/Blood_Banking_and_Blood_Products_Market_Report.asp

Gordenker, Leon (1995) *International Cooperation in Response to AIDS*. London: Pinter.

Gostin, Lawrence O. (2008) 'Meeting basic survival needs of the world's least healthy people: toward a framework convention on global health', *Georgetown Law Journal*, 96, 331–92.

Gostin, Lawrence O., Gorik Ooms, Mark Heywood et al. (2010) 'The Joint Action and Learning Initiative on National and Global Responsibilities for Health', World Health Report Background Paper No. 53. Available at: http://www.who.int/healthsystems/topics/financing/healthreport/JALI_No53.pdf.

Grace, Cheri (2010) *Product Development Partnerships (PDPs): Lessons from PDPs Established to Develop New Health Technologies for Neglected Diseases*. London: DfID.

Graham, Bob (2008) *World at Risk: The Report of the Commission on the Prevention of WMD Proliferation and Terrorism*. New York: Vintage.

Graham, David T. and Nana Poku (eds.) (2000), *Migration, Globalisation and Human Security*. London: Routledge.

Greenhalgh, Trisha (1997) 'How to read a paper: Papers that summarise other papers (systematic reviews and meta-analyses)', *British Medical Journal*, 215, 672.

Grüning, Thilo, Heide Weishaar, Jeff Collin and Anna B. Gilmore (2011) 'Tobacco industry attempts to influence and use the German government to undermine the WHO Framework Convention on Tobacco Control', *Tobacco Control*. Available at: http://tobaccocontrol.bmj.com/content/early/2011/06/09/tc.2010.042093.abstract

Haggett, Peter (2000) *The Geographical Structure of Epidemics*. Oxford: Oxford University Press.

Ham, Chris (1997) *Health Care Reform: Learning from International Experience*. Buckingham: Open University Press.

Harrabin, Roger, Anne Coote and Jessica Allen (2003) *Health in the News: Risk, Reporting and Media Influence*. London: The King's Fund.

Harris, Stuart (2004) 'Marrying foreign policy and health: feasible or doomed to fail?', *Medical Journal of Australia*, 180(4), 171–3.

Heinccken, Lindy (2003) 'Facing a merciless enemy: HIV/AIDS and the South African armed forces', *Armed Forces and Society*, 29(2), 281–300.

Held, David, Anthony McGrew, David Goldblatt and Jonathan Perraton (1999) *Global Transformations, Politics, Economics and Culture*. Stanford, CA: Stanford University Press.

Hoffman, Steven J. (2010) 'The evolution, etiology and eventualities of the global health security regime', *Health Policy and Planning*, 25(6), 510–22.

Hogan, Helen and Andy Haines (2011) 'Global health: a positive addition to public health training?', *Journal of Public Health*, 33(2), 317–18.

Hollis, Martin and Steve Smith (1991) *Explaining and Understanding International Relations*. Oxford: Oxford University Press.

Hotez, Peter J. (2008) 'Training the next generation of global health scientists: a school of appropriate technology for global health', *PloS Neglected Tropical Diseases*, 2(8). Available at: http://www.plosntds.org/article/info%3Adoi%2F10.1371%2Fjournal.pntd.0000279.

Hunt, Paul (2006) 'The human right to the highest attainable standard of health: New opportunities and challenges', *Transactions of the Royal Society of Tropical Medicine and Hygiene*, 100(7), 603–7.

Huysmans, Jeff (1997) 'Revisiting Copenhagen, or, About the creative development of a security studies agenda in Europe', *European Journal of International Relations*, 4(4), 488–506.

IAVI [International AIDS Vaccine Initiative] (2010) *Innovative Product Development Partnerships*, Policy Brief No. 26. Available at: http://www.iavi.org/Lists/IAVIPublications/attachments/eb7b4247-6816-4094-9f54-9f2f2b99e95a/IAVI_Innovative_Product_Development_Partnerships_2010_ENG.pdf.

ICG [International Crisis Group] (2001) *HIV/AIDS as a Security Issue*. Brussels: ICG.

IMAP (2010) *Pharmaceuticals and Biotech Industry Global Report – 2011*. Delaware. Available at: http://www.imap.com/imap/media/resources/IMAP_Pharma Report_8_272B8752E0FB3.pdf

IMS (2011) 'Institute for Healthcare Informatics, IMS Institute forecasts global spending on medicines to reach nearly \$1.1 trillion by 2015', Press Release, 11 May. Available at: http://www.imshealth.com/portal/site/ imshealth/menuitem.a46c6d4df3db4b3d88f611019418c22a/?vgnextoid= 01146b46f9aff210VgnVCM100000ed152ca2RCRD&vgnextchannel=b5e57 900b55a5110VgnVCM10000071812ca2RCRD&vgnextfmt=default.

Ingram, Alan (2007) 'HIV/AIDS, security and the geo-politics of US-Nigerian relations', *Review of International Political Economy*, 14(3), 510–34.

Ingram, Alan (2010) 'Governmentality and security in the US President's Emergency Plan for AIDS Relief (PEPFAR)', *Geoforum*, 41, 607–16. Available at: http://www.sciencedirect.com/science/article/pii/S0016718510000242.

Institute of Medicine (US) (1997) *America's Vital Interest in Global Health*. Washington, DC: National Academy Press.

Jacobson, Harold K. (1974) 'WHO: Medicine, regionalism, and managed politics', in R.W. Cox, H.K. Jacobson, et al. *The Anatomy of Influence, Decision Making in International Organization*. New Haven, CT: Yale University Press.

Jain, Sagar C. (1991) 'Global health: Emerging frontier of international health', *Asia-Pacific Journal of Public Health*, 5(2), 112–14.

Jamison, Dean T., W. Henry Mosley, Anthony R. Measham and Jose Luis Bobadilla (eds.) (1993) *Disease Priorities in Developing Countries*, 2nd edn. Washington, DC: World Bank.

Jamison, Dean T., Julio Frenk and Felicia Knaul (1998) 'International collective action in health: objectives, functions and rationale', *Lancet*, 351, 514–17.

Janes, Craig R. and Kitty K. Corbett (2009) 'Anthropology and global health', *Annual Review of Anthropology*, 38, 167–83.

Janes, Craig R. and Kitty K. Corbett (2011) 'Global health', in P.I. Erickson and M. Singer (eds.) *A Companion Guide to Medical Anthropology*. New York: John Wiley & Sons.

Jones, Keri-Ann (2010) 'New complexities and approaches to global health diplomacy: View from the US Department of State', *PLoS Medicine*, 7(5). Available at: http://www.plosmedicine.org/article/info%3Adoi%2 F10.1371%2Fjournal.pmed.1000276.

Jones, R.J. Barry (1995), *Globalisation and Interdependence in the International Political Economy*. London: Pinter.

Justice Africa (2004) 'HIV/AIDS and the threat to security in Africa', submission to the UN Secretary General's High-Level Panel on Threats, Challenges and Change, 2 May, Addis Ababa.

Kaiser Family Foundation (2011) 'The US Government's Global Health Policy Architecture: Structure, Programs and Funding', (#7881), June. Available at: http://www.kff.org/globalhealth/7881.cfm

Kamradt-Scott, Adam (in press) 'The International Health Regulations 2005: A case study in global health diplomacy', in T. Novotny, H. Feldbaum and

I. Kickbusch (eds.) *Twenty-First Century Health Diplomacy*. Singapore: World Scientific Press.

Kamradt-Scott, Adam and Kelley Lee (2011) 'Global health security interrupted: The World Health Organisation, Indonesia and H5N1', *Political Studies*, 59(4), 831–47.

Kanchanachitra, Churnrurtai, Magnus Lindelow, Timothy Johnston et al. (2011) 'Human resources for health in southeast Asia: shortages, distributional challenges, and international trade in health services', *Lancet*, 377(9767), 769–81.

Kanji, Najmi, Nazneen Kanji and Firoze Manji (1991) 'From development to sustained crisis: Structural adjustment, equity and health', *Social Science and Medicine*, 33(9), 985–93.

Kassalow, Jordan S. (2001) *Why Health is Important to US Foreign Policy*. New York: Council on Foreign Relations.

Kates, Jennifer, Julie Fischer and Eric Lief (2009) *The US Government's Global Health Policy Architecture: Structure, Programs, and Funding*. Washington, DC: The Henry Kaiser Family Foundation.

Kates, Jennifer, Carlos Avila, Benjamin Gobet, Eric Leif and Adam Wexler (2011) *Financing the Response to AIDS in Low- and Middle-Income Countries: International Assistance from Donor Governments in 2010*. Washington, DC: Kaiser Family Foundation/UNAIDS Available at: http://www.kff.org/hivaids/upload/7347-07.pdf.

Kegley, Charles W. and Eugene R. Wittkopf (1989) *World Politics: Trend and Transformation*, 3rd edn. New York: St Martin's Press.

Keohane, Robert O. (1984) *After Hegemony: Cooperation and Discord in the World Political Economy*. Princeton, NJ: Princeton University Press.

Keohane, Robert O. and Joseph S. Nye (1977) *Power and Interdependence: World Politics in Transition*. Boston, MA: Little, Brown and Company.

Kerry Vanessa B. and Kelley Lee (2007) 'TRIPS, the Doha Declaration and Paragraph 6 decision: What are the remaining steps for protecting access to medicines?', *Globalization and Health*, 3(3). Available at: http://www.globalizationandhealth.com/content/3/1/3.

Kickbusch, Ilona and Graham Lister (eds.) (2006) *European Perspectives on Global Health: A Policy Glossary*. Brussels: European Commission.

Kirton, John (2009) 'Introduction', in J. Kirton (ed.) *Global Health*. New York: Ashgate.

Knox, Richard (2011) 'WHO resolves impasse over sharing of flu viruses, access to vaccines'. Available at: http://sanevax.org/news-blog/2011/04/who-resolves-impasse-over-sharing-of-flu-viruses-access-to-vaccines/.

Koplan, Jeffrey P., T. Christopher Bond, Michael H. Merson et al. (2009) 'Towards a common definition of global health', *Lancet*, 373, 1993–5.

KPMG (2011) *Issues Monitor: Medical Tourism Gaining Momentum*. London, May. Available at: http://www.kpmg.com/Global/en/IssuesAndInsights/Articles Publications/Issues-monitor-healthcare/Documents/issues-monitor-healthcare-may-2011.pdf.

Kristiansen, Ivar S. and Gavin Mooney (eds.) (2004), *Evidence-Based Medicine: In Its Place*. Abingdon: Routledge.

Kumaranayake, Lilani and Sally Lake (2002) 'Regulation in the context of Global Health Markets', in K. Lee, K. Buse and S. Fustukian (eds.) *Health Policy in the Globalising World*. Cambridge: Cambridge University Press.

Kurki, Milja and Colin Wight (2007) 'International Relations and social science', in T. Dunne, M. Kurki and S. Smith (eds.) *International Relations Theories*. Oxford: Oxford University Press.

Labonte, Ronald (2004) 'Nailing health planks into the foreign policy platform: the Canadian experience', *Medical Journal of Australia*, 180(4), 159–62.

Labonte, Ronald and Michelle L. Gagnon (2010) 'Framing health and foreign policy: Lessons for global health diplomacy', *Globalization and Health*, 6(14). Available at: http://www.globalizationandhealth.com/content/6/1/14.

Larson, James S. (1999) 'The conceptualization of health', *Medical Care Research and Review*, 56(2), 123–36.

Leach, Melissa and Sarah Dry (2010) 'Epidemic narratives', in S. Dry and M. Leach, *Epidemics: Science, Governance and Social Justice*. Abingdon: Earthscan.

Leach, Melissa, Ian Scoones and Andrew Stirling (2010) 'Governing epidemics in an age of complexity: Narratives, politics and pathways to sustainability', *Global Environmental Change*, 20(3), 369–77.

Leary, Virginia A. (1994), 'The right to health in international human rights law', *Health and Human Rights*, 1(1), 24–56.

Lederman, Doug (2009) 'Boom in global health studies', *Inside Higher Education*, 14 September. Available at: http://www.insidehighered.com/news/2009/09/14/health.

Lee, Andrew C.K., Jennifer A. Hall and Kate L. Mandeville (2011) 'Global public health training in the UK: Preparing for the future', *Journal of Public Health*, 33(2), 310–16.

Lee, Kelley (2000) 'Globalisation and health policy: A review of the literature and proposed research and policy agenda', in A. Bambas, J.A. Casas, H.A. Drayton and A. Valdes (eds.) *Health and Human Development in the New Global Economy*. Washington, DC: Pan American Health Organization.

Lee, Kelley (2003) *Globalization and Health: An Introduction*. Basingstoke: Macmillan.

Lee, Kelley (2004) 'The pit and the pendulum: Can globalization take health governance forward?', *Development*, 47(2), 11–17.

Lee, Kelley (2010) 'International organization and health/disease', in K. Stiles (ed.) *International Studies Compendium*. London: Wiley-Blackwell.

Lee, Kelley and Eduardo J. Gomez (2011) 'Brazil's ascendance: the soft power role of global health diplomacy', *European Business Review*, 10 January. Available at: http://www.europeanbusinessreview.com/?p=3400.

Lee, Kelley and Richard D. Smith (in press) 'What is 'global health diplomacy'? A conceptual review', *Global Health Governance*.

Lee, Kelley, Luis Carlos Chagas and Thomas E. Novotny (2010) 'Brazil and the Framework Convention on Tobacco Control: Global health diplomacy as soft power', *PLoS Medicine*, 7(4). Available at: http://www.plosmedicine. org/article/info%3Adoi%2F10.1371%2Fjournal.pmed.1000232.

Legge, David (2005) 'Health inequalities in the new world order', People's Health Assembly, Issue Papers. Available at: http://www.phmovement.org/ pha2000/presentations/legge.html.

Lesser, Lenard I. , Cara B. Ebbeling, Merrill Goozner, David Wypij and David S. Ludwig (2007) 'Relationship between funding source and conclusion among nutrition-related scientific articles', *PLoS Medicine*, 4(1). Available at: http://www.plosmedicine.org/article/info:doi/10.1371/journal.pmed. 0040005.

Leutwyler, Kristin (2000) 'Academic credibility vs. industry cash', *Scientific American*, 1 November. Available at http://www.scientificamerican.com/ article.cfm?id=academic-credibility-vs-i.

Lexchin, Joel, Lisa A. Bero, Benjamin Djulbegovic and Otavio Clark (2003) 'Pharmaceutical industry sponsorship and research outcome and quality: systematic review', *British Medical Journal*, 326(7400), 1167–70.

Lin, ching-Fu (2011) 'Global food safety: exploring key elements for an international regulatory strategy', *Virginia Journal of International Law*, 51(3), 637–95. Available at: http://www.vjil.org/assets/pdfs/vol51/issue3/Lin. pdf.

Loewenson, Rene (1993) 'Structural adjustment and health policy in Africa', *International Journal of Health Services*, 23(4), 717–40.

Loewenson, Rene (2001) 'Globalization and occupational health: a perspective from southern Africa', *Bulletin of the World Health Organization*, 79(9), 863–8.

London, Leslie and Helen Schneider (2011) 'Globalisation and health inequalities: Can a human rights paradigm create space for civil society action?', *Social Science and Medicine*, 3(6). Available at: http://www.science-direct.com/science/article/pii/S0277953611001857.

Lucas, Adetokunbo (1998) 'WHO at country level', *Lancet*, 351(9104), 743–7.

Lugalla, Joe L.P. (1995) 'The impact of structural adjustment policies on women's and children's health in Tanzania', *Review of African Political Economy*, 22(63), 43–53.

Lundh, Andreas, Marika Barbateskovic, Asbjorn Hrobjartsson and Peter C. Gotzsche (2010) 'Conflicts of interest at medical journals: the influence of industry-supported randomised trials on journal impact factors and revenue – cohort study', *PLoS Medicine*, 7(10). Available at: http://www. plosmedicine.org/article/info%3Adoi%2F10.1371%2Fjournal.pmed. 1000354.

Lynn, Laurence E. (1998) 'A critical analysis of the new public management', *International Public Management Journal*, 1(1), 107–23.

McCoy, David, Sudeep Chand and Devi Sridhar (2009) 'Global health funding: How much, where it comes from and where it goes', *Health Policy and Planning* 24(6), 407–17.

McCoy, David, Gayatri Kembhavi, Jinesh Patel and Akish Luintel (2010) 'The Bill and Melinda Gates Foundation's grant-making programme for global health', *Lancet*, 373(9675), 1645–53.

Macfarlane Sarah B., Marian Jacobs and Ephata E. Kaaya (2008) 'In the name of global health: trends in academic institutions', *Journal of Public Health Policy*, 29(4), 383–401.

McInnes, Colin (2006) 'HIV/AIDS and security', *International Affairs*, 82(2), 315–26.

McInnes, Colin (2007) 'HIV/AIDS and national security' in N. Poku et al. (eds.), *Governing a Pandemic*. Aldershot: Ashgate.

McInnes, Colin and Kelley Lee (2006) 'Health, security and foreign policy', *Review of International Studies*, 32(1), 5–23.

McInnes, Colin and Simon Rushton (2010) 'HIV, AIDS and security: Where are we now?', *International Affairs*, 86(1), 225–45.

McLean, Thomas R. (2009) 'The global market for healthcare: Economics and regulation', *Wisconsin International Law Journal*, 26(3), 591–645.

McMichael, Anthony J. and Robert Beaglehole (2000) 'The changing global context of public health', *Lancet*, 356, 495–9.

Manning, Nick (2001) 'The legacy of the New Public Management in developing countries', *International Review of Administrative Sciences*, 67, 297–312.

Markel, Howard and Alexandra M. Stern (2002) 'The foreignness of germs: The persistent association of immigrants and disease in American society', *Milbank Quarterly*, 80(4), 757–88.

Marmot, Michael (2007) 'Achieving health equity: from root causes to fair outcomes', *Lancet*, 370(9593), 1153–63.

Martinson, Brian C., Melissa S. Anderson and Raymond de Vries (2005) 'Scientists behaving badly', *Nature*, 435, 737–8.

May, Christopher (2009) *The Global Political Economy of Intellectual Property Rights: The New Enclosures*, 2nd edn. London: Routledge.

Maynard, Alan (ed.) (2005) *The Public-Private Mix for Health*. Milton Keynes: Radcliffe.

Mearsheimer, John J. (2001) *The Tragedy of Great Power Politics*. New York: W.W. Norton.

Médecins Sans Frontières (2003) *Doha Derailed: A Progress Report on TRIPS and Access to Medicines*, Campaign for Access to Essential Medicines. Available at: http://www.msfaccess.org/sites/default/files/MSF_assets/Access/Docs/ACCESS_report_DohaDerailed_ENG_2003.pdf.

Mejia, Raul, Veronica Schoj, Joaquin Barnoya, Maria Laura Flores and Eliseo J. Perez-Stable (2008) 'Tobacco industry strategies to obstruct the FCTC in Argentina', *CVD Prevention and Control*, 3(4): 173–9.

Mello, Michelle M., Brian R. Clarridge and David M. Studdart (2005) 'Academic medical centers' standards for clinical-trial agreements with industry', *New England Journal of Medicine*, 352, 2202–10.

Michler, Inga (2011) 'A human-waste gold mine: Bill Gates looks to reinvent the toilet', *Time*, 13 July. Available at: http://www.time.com/time/world/article/0,8599,2082509,00.html.

Møgedal, Sigrun and Benedikte Louise Alveberg (2010) 'Can foreign policy make a difference to health?', *PLoS Medicine*, 7(5). Available at: http://www.plosmedicine.org/article/info:doi/10.1371/journal.pmed.1000274.

Mohan, John (1991) 'The internationalisation and commercialisation of health care in Britain', *Environment and Planning*, 23(6), 853–67.

Moon, Suerie, Nicole A. Szlezak, Catherine M. Michaud et al. (2010) 'The global health system: Lessons for a stronger institutional framework', *PLoS Medicine*, 7(1). Available at: http://www.plosmedicine.org/article/info%3Adoi%2F10.1371%2Fjournal.pmed.1000193.

Moore, Harriet (2008) 'Contagion from Abroad: US Press Framing of Immigrants and Epidemics, 1891 to 1893', MA Thesis, Department of Communication, Georgia State University. Available at: http://digitalarchive.gsu.edu/communication_theses/42/.

Moran, Mary, Javier Guzman, Anne-Laure Ropars et al. (2008) *Neglected Disease Research and Development: How Much Are We Really Spending?* Sydney: George Institute for International Health.

Muggli, Monique E., Kelley Lee, Quan Gan, Jon O. Ebbert and Richard D. Hurt (2008) 'Efforts to reprioritise the agenda in China: British American Tobacco's actions to divert health policy from secondhand smoke to liver disease prevention', *PLoS Medicine*, 5(12). Available at: http://www.plosmedicine.org/article/info:doi/10.1371/journal.pmed.0050251.

Murray, Christopher J.L. and Julio Frenk (2010) 'Ranking 37th – Measuring the performance of the US health care system', *New England Journal of Medicine*, 362(2), 98–99.

Murray, Christopher J.L. and Alan D. Lopez (1996) 'Evidence-based health policy – Lessons from the Global Burden of Disease Study', *Science*, 1 November.

Navarro, Vicente (1982) 'The labor process and health: A historical materialist interpretation', *International Journal of Health Services*, 12(1), 5–29.

Navarro, Vicente and Carlos Muntaner (eds.) (2004) *Political and Economic Determinants of Population Health and Well-being: Controversies and Developments.* Amityville, NY: Baywood Publishing.

Nestle, Marion (2003) *Food Politics: How the Food Industry Influences Nutrition and Health.* Berkeley, CA: University of California Press.

Neumayer, Eric (2004) 'Arab-related bilateral and multilateral sources of development finance: Issues, trends and the way forward', *The World Economy*, 27(2), 281–300.

Ng, Nora Y. and Jennifer Ruger (2010) 'Emerging and transitioning countries' role in global health', *St. Louis University Journal of Health Law and Policy*, 3, 253–89.

NIC [US National Intelligence Council] (2008) *Strategic Implications of Global Health.* Available at: http://www.dni.gov/nic/NIC_specialproducts.html.

Nishtar, Sania (2004) 'Public–private "partnerships" in health – a global call to action', *Health Research Policy and Systems*, 2, 5.

Novotny, Thomas and Ilona Kickbusch (2009) 'Global health diplomacy – a bridge to innovative collaborative action', *Global Forum for Health Research*,

5. Available at: http://light.globalforumhealth.org/Media-Publications/Publications/Global-Forum-Update-on-Research-for-Health-Volume-5-Fostering-innovation-for-global-health/Global-Forum-Update-on-Research-for-Health-Volume-5-Fostering-innovation-for-global-health-Individual-articles.

Nye, Joseph S. (1988) 'Neorealism and neoliberalism', *World Politics*, 40(2), 235–51.

Nye, Joseph S. (1990) *Bound to Lead: the Changing Nature of American Power*. New York: Basic Books.

Nye, Joseph S. (2009) 'Get smart: combining hard and soft power', *Foreign Affairs*, 88(4), 160–3.

Ogata, Sadako and Jonathan Cels (2003) 'Human security – protecting and empowering the people', *Global Governance*, 9, 273–82.

Ogata, Sadako and Amartya Sen (2003) *Human Security Now: Commission on Human Security*. New York: Commission on Human Security.

Oomman, Nandini, Michael Bernstein and Steven Rosenzweig (2007) *Following the Funding for HIV/AIDS, A comparative analysis of the funding practices of PEPFAR, the Global Fund and World Bank MAP in Mozambique, Uganda and Zambia*. Washington, DC: Centre for Global Development. Available at: http://allafrica.com/download/resource/main/main/idatcs/00011395:3f2a0f1cddef4aaec2e61c2fe9018885.pdf.

Ong, Elisa K. and Stanton A. Glantz (2000) 'Tobacco industry efforts subverting International Agency for Research on Cancer's second-hand smoke study', *Lancet*, 355, 1253–9.

Onuf, Nicholas (1989) *A World of our Making: Rules and Rule in Social Theory and International Relations*. Columbia SC: University of South Carolina Press.

Organisation for Economic Cooperation and Development [OECD] (2005) *Health Technology and Decision Making*. Paris: OECD.

Organization for Economic Cooperation and Development [OECD] (2011) *Health Indicators at a Glance 2011*. Paris: OECD.

Organisation for Economic Cooperation and Development [OECD] (2012), *Aid Statistics*. Available at: http://www.oecd.org/document/49/0,3746,en_2649_34447_46582641_1_1_1_1,00.html

Oslo Declaration (2007) 'Oslo Ministerial Declaration – global health: a pressing foreign policy issue of our time', *Lancet*, 369, 1373–8.

Oxfam (2011) Available at: http://www.oxfam.org.uk/applications/blogs/scotland/2011/04/gleneagles_aid_commitments_mis.html.

Ozdemir, Vural, Don Husereau, S. Hyland, S. Samper and Mohd Zuki Salleh (2009) 'Personalized medicine beyond genomics: new technologies, global health diplomacy and anticipatory governance', *Current Pharmacogenomics and Personalized Medicine*, 7(4), 225–30.

Panosian, Clare and Thomas J. Coates (2006) 'The new medical "missionaries" – Grooming the next generation of global health workers', *New England Journal of Medicine*, 354, 1771–3.

Paris, Roland (2001) 'Human security: paradigm shift or hot air?', *International Security*, 26(2), 87–102.

Parker, Tracy (2011) *THA Overview*, Canada-US Collaborations on Health and Biosecurity, Washington, DC: Office of Health Affairs. Available at: www.pbphpc.org/wp-content/.../07/OHA-Overview_June-2011.pdf.

Pauwelyn, Joost (2010) 'The dog that barked but didn't bite: 15 years of intellectual property disputes at the WTO', *Journal of International Dispute Settlement*, 1(2), 389–429.

Petticrew, Mark (2001) 'Systematic reviews from astronomy to zoology: myths and misconceptions', *British Medical Journal*, 322(7278), 98–101.

Petticrew, Mark (2011) 'When are complex interventions "complex"? When are simple interventions "simple"?', *European Journal of Public Health*, 21(4), 397–8.

Pilcavage, Christine (forthcoming) 'Japan's ODA and global health governance', in K. Lee, T. Pang and Y. Tang (eds.) *Asia's Role in Global Health Governance*. London: Routledge.

Plotnikova, Evgeniya Vadimovna (2011) 'Cross-border mobility of health professionals: Contesting patients' rights to health', *Social Science and Medicine* (online only). Available at: http://www.sciencedirect.com/science/article/pii/S0277953611000980.

Pogge, Thomas W. (2005) 'Human rights and global health: a research program', *Metaphilosophy*, 36(1/2), 182–208.

Pollock, Allyson M. (2004) *NHS plc*. London: Verso.

Pollock, Allyson M. and David Price (2000) 'Rewriting the regulations: How the World Trade Organisation could accelerate privatization in health-care systems', *Lancet*, 356, 1995–2000.

Porter, Michael E. (2009) 'A strategy for health care reform – Toward a value-based system', *New England Journal of Medicine*, 361, 109–12.

Powell, Colin L. (2004) 'Presentation at HIV/AIDS plenary', 22 September 2003. Available at: http://www.state.gov.

Prabhu, K.Seeta (1994) 'World Development Report 1993: Structural adjustment and the health sector in India', *Social Scientist*, 22(9), 89–97.

Prescott, Elizabeth (2003) 'SARS: a warning', *Survival*, 45(3), 207–26.

Price-Smith, Andrew (2002) *The Health of Nations: Infectious Disease, Environmental Change and Their Effects on National Security and Development*. Cambridge, MA: MIT Press.

Quam, Lois (1989) 'Post-war American health care: The many costs of market failure', *Oxford Review of Economic Policy*, 5(1), 113–23.

Rajaratnam, Julie Knoll, Jake R. Marcus, Alison Levin-Rector et al. (2010) 'Worldwide mortality in men and women aged 15–59 years from 1970 to 2010: A systematic analysis', *Lancet*, 375(9727), 1704–20.

Ramiah, Ilavenil and Michael R. Reich (2005) 'Public-private partnerships and antiretroviral drugs for HIV/AIDS: Lessons from Botswana', *Health Affairs*, 24(2), 545–51.

Reeves, Margaret and Suzanne Brundage (2011) *Leveraging the World Health Organization's Core Strengths*. Washington, DC: Center for Strategic and International Studies.

Ring, Ian and Ngaire Brown (2003) 'The health status of indigenous populations and others', *British Medical Journal*, 372, 404. Available at: http://www.bmj.com/content/327/7412/404.full.

Robertson, Roland (1992) *Globalization, Social Theory and Global Culture*. London: Sage.

Rodier, Guenael (2007) 'New rules on international public health security', *Bulletin of the World Health Organization*, 85(6), 428–30.

Rodier, Guenael, Allison L. Greenspan, James M. Highes and David L. Heymann (2007) 'Global public health security', *Emerging Infectious Diseases*, 13(10), 1447–52.

Romanow, Roy, J. (2002) *Building on Values: The Future of Health Care in Canada*, Final Report of Commission on the Future of Health Care in Canada (the Romanow Commission). Available at: http://www.healthcarecommissoin.ca.

Rose, Andrew (2005) 'Which international institutions promote international trade?', *Review of International Economics*, 13(4): 682–98.

Rowe, Sylvia, Nick Alexander, Fergus M. Clydesdale, Rhona S. Applebaum, Stephanie Atkinson et al. (2009) 'Funding food science and nutrition research: Financial conflicts and scientific integrity', *American Journal of Clinical Nutrition*, 89(1), 285–91.

Ruger, Jennifer P. and Hak-Ju Kim (2006) 'Global health inequalities: An international comparison', *Journal of Epidemiology and Community Health*, 60, 928–936.

Ruger, Jennifer and Derek Yach (2005) 'Global functions at the World Health Organization', *British Medical Journal*, 330, 1099–100.

Ruggie, John (1998) *Constructing the World Polity*. London: Routledge.

Sachs, Jeffrey D. (2004) 'Health in the developing world: achieving the Millennium Development Goals', *Bulletin of the World Health Organization*, 82(12), 947–9.

Samet, Jonathan M. and Thomas A. Burke (2001) 'Turning science into junk: The tobacco industry and passive smoking', *American Journal of Public Health*, 91(11), 1742–4.

Scholte, Jan Aart (2000) *Globalization: A Critical Introduction*. London: Palgrave Macmillan.

Seigel, Karen R., Andrea B. Feigl, Sandeep P. Kishore and David Stuckler (2011) 'Misalignment between perceptions and actual global burden of disease: Evidence from the US population', *Global Health Action*, 4, 6339.

Sell, Susan K. (2003) 'Trade issues and international law', *Emory International Law Review*, 17(2), 933–54.

Sen, Amartya (2000) 'Why human security?', text of presentation at the International Symposium on Human Security, Tokyo, 28 July. Available at: http://www.humansecurity-chs.org/activities/outreach/Sen2000.pdf.

Sen, Kasturi and Meri Koivusalso (1998) 'Health care reforms and developing countries – a critical overview', *International Journal of Health Planning and Management*, 13(3), 199–215.

Shiffman, Jeremy (2006) 'Donor funding priorities for communicable disease control in the developing world', *Health Policy and Planning*, 21(6), 411–20.

Shiffman, Jeremy (2008) 'Has donor prioritization of HIV/AIDS displaced aid for other health issues?', *Health Policy and Planning*, 23(2), 95–100.

Shobert Benjamin (2012) 'New China FDI rules put focus on ascent', *Asia Times*, 24 January.

Siddiqi, Javed (1995) *World Health and World Politics, The World Health Organization and the U.N. System*. London: Hurst & Company.

Silberschmidt, Gaudenz, Don Matheson and Ilona Kickbusch (2008) 'Creating a Committee C of the World Health Assembly', *Lancet* 371, 1483–6.

Sinha, Kounteya (2011) 'Global consensus to share influenza virus samples', *The Times of India*, 19 April.

Sjostedt, Roxanna (2010) 'Health issues and securitization: the construction of HIV/AIDS as a US national security threat', in T. Balzacq, *Securitization Theory: How Security Problems Emerge and Dissolve*. New York: Routledge.

Smith, Frank (2010) 'The false promise of global governance during transnational outbreaks?', unpublished paper presented at the International Studies Association Annual Convention, New Orleans.

Smith, Richard D., Kelley Lee and Nick Drager (2009) 'Trade and health: An agenda for action', *Lancet*, 373(9665), 768–73.

Smith, Steve (2001) 'Reflectivist and constructivist approaches', in J. Baylis and S. Smith (eds.) *Globalization of World Politics*, 2nd edn. Oxford: Oxford University Press.

Smith, Steve (2007) 'Diversity and disciplinarity in International Relations', in T. Dunne, M. Kurki and S. Smith (eds.) *International Relations Theories*. Oxford: Oxford University Press.

Spicer, Neil and Aisling Walsh (2011) '10 best resources on . . . the current effects of global health initiatives on country health systems', *Health Policy and Planning*, published online at doi:10.1093/heapol/czr034.

Sridhar, Devi, Stephen J. Morrison and Peter Piot (2011) 'Getting the politics right for the 2011 UN High-Level Meeting on Non-Communicable Diseases', Washington, DC: CSIS.

Stocker, Karen, Howard Waitzkin and Celia Iriart (1999) 'The exportation of managed care to Latin America', *New England Journal of Medicine*, 340, 1131–6.

Stopford, John and Susan Strange (1991) *Rival States, Rival Firms: Competition for World Market Shares*. Cambridge: Cambridge University Press.

Strange, Susan (1998) *States and Markets*, 2nd edn. London: Continuum.

Strongin, Robin and C. Stephen Redhead (2001) *Bioterrorism: Summary of a CRS/National Health Policy Forum Seminar on Federal, State and Local Public*

Health Preparedness, Congressional Research Service [CRS] Report for Congress. Washington, DC: CRS.

Stuckler, David, Sanjay Basu and Martin McKee (2011a) 'Global health philanthropy and institutional relationships: How should conflicts of interest be addressed?', *PloS Medicine*, 8(4). Available at: http://www.plosmedicine.org/article/info:doi/10.1371/journal.pmed.1001020.

Stuckler, David, Sanjay Basu and Martin McKee (2011b) 'Health care capacity and allocations among South Africa's provinces: Infrastructure-inequality traps after the end of apartheid', *American Journal of Public Health*, 101(1), 165–72.

Stuckler, David, Sanjay Basu, Stephanie W. Wang and Martin McKee (2011c) 'Does recession reduce global health aid? Evidence from 15 high income countries, 1975–2007', *Bulletin of the World Health Organization*, 89(4), 252–7. Available at: http://www.who.int/bulletin/volumes/89/4/10-080663.pdf.

Summer, L. (2011) 'Integration, concentration and competition in the provider marketplace', AcademyHealth. Available at: http://www.academyhealth.org/files/publications/AH_R_Integration%20FINAL2.pdf

Surel, Yves (2000) 'The role of cognitive and normative frames in policy-making', *Journal of European Public Policy*, 7(4), 495–512.

Susser, Mervyn (1993) 'Health as a human right: an epidemiologist's perspective on the public health', *American Journal of Public Health*, 83(3), 418–26.

Tadros, Mariz (2010) 'Scapepigging: H1N1 Influenza in Egypt', in S. Dry and M. Leach (eds.) *Epidemics: Science, Governance and Social Justice*. Abingdon: Earthscan.

Tarabusi, Claudio C. and GrahamVickery (1998) 'Globalization in the pharmaceutical industry, Part 1', *International Journal of Health Services*, 28(1), 67–105.

Thomas, Caroline (2000) *Global Governance, Development and Human Security: The Challenge of Poverty and Inequality*. London: Pluto.

Thomas, Caroline and Martin Weber (2004) 'The politics of global health governance: Whatever happened to "health for all by the year 2000"?' *Global Governance*, 10(2), 187–205.

Thompson, Tommy G. (2005) 'The cure for tyranny' (editorial), *The Boston Globe*, 24 October. Available at: www.boston.com/news/globe/editorial_opinion/oped/articles/2005/10/24/the_cure_for_tyranny/.

Toebes, Brigit (1999) 'Towards an improved understanding of the international human right to health', *Human Rights Quarterly*, 21(3), 661–79.

Turner, Leigh (2007) 'First world healthcare at third world prices: Globalization, bioethics and medical tourism', *BioSocieties*, 2, 303–25.

UC [University of California] (no date a) *Atlas of Global Inequality, Causes of death*. Available at: http://ucatlas.ucsc.edu/cause.php.

UC (no date b) *Atlas of Global Inequality, Health Care Spending*. Available at: http://ucatlas.ucsc.edu/spend.php.

ul-Haq, Mahbub (1995) *Reflections on Human Development*. Oxford: Oxford University Press.

UN (2009) World Population Ageing Report, United Nations Department of Economic and Social Affairs/Population Division).

UN (no date) Millennium Development Goals. Available at: http://www.un.org/millenniumgoals/global.shtml

UNAIDS [United Nations Joint Programme on HIV/AIDS] (2003) *On the Front Line: A Review of the Policies and Programmes to address HIV/AIDS among Peacekeepers and Uniformed Personnel.* Geneva/New York: UNAIDS.

UNAIDS (2005) *AIDS Epidemic Update: December 2005.* Geneva/New York: UNAIDS.

UNAIDS (2008) 'HIV-related travel conditions', 4 March. Available at: http://www.unaids.org/en/Resources/PressCentre/Featurestories/2008/March/20080304HIVrelatedtravelrestrictions/.

UNDP [United Nations Development Programme] (1990) *Human Development Report 1990.* Available at: http://hdr.undp.org/en/media/hdr_1990_en_front.pdf.

UNDP (1994) *Human Development Report: New Dimensions of Human Security.* New York: Oxford University Press.

UNGA [United Nations General Assembly] (2010) *Global Health and Foreign Policy: Note by the Secretary General,* A/65/399. New York: United Nations.

UNGA (2011) *Prevention and control of non-communicable diseases: Report of the Secretary-General,* A/66/8. New York: United Nations.

UNSC [Security Council] (2000a) *UN Security Council Press Release SC/6781,* 10 January. Available at: http://www.un.org/News/Press/docs/2000/20000110.sc6781.doc.html.

UNSC (2000b) *Resolution 1308 on the responsibility of the Security Council in the maintenance of international peace and security: HIV/AIDS and international peacekeeping operations.* Available at: http://www.un.org/Docs/sc/unsc_resolutions.html.

UNDP KO [Department of Peace Keeping Operations] (2005) *Background Note: 31 December 2005.* Available at: http://www.un.org/Depts/dpko/bnote.htm#unmil.

UN High Level Panel (2004) *A More Secure World: Report of the Secretary-General's High Level Panel on Threats, Challenges and Change.* Available at: http://www.un.org/secureworld/report2.pdf.

UN Secretariat (2003) *The Impact of AIDS,* Report by the Population Division, Department of Economic and Social Affairs, 2 September, New York: United Nations.

USAID (no date) 'About USAID'. Available at: http://www.usaid.gov/about_usaid/.

US Congressional Budget Office (2007) *Federal Support for Research and Development.* Washington, DC: US Congress.

US Department of Health and Human Services, Centers for Disease Control and Prevention [CDC] (2011) 'Health Disparities and Inequalities Report', *Morbidity and Mortality Weekly Report,* 60 (Supplement). Atlanta: US Department of Health and Human Services. Available at: http://www.cdc.gov/mmwr/pdf/other/su6001.pdf

US Joint Forces Command (2010) *The Joint Operating Environment 2010, Ready for Today, Preparing for Tomorrow*. Available at: www.ndu.edu/pinnacle/doc-Uploaded/JOE%202010%20FINAL.pdf.

US State Department (1999) *United States Strategic Plan for International Affairs*, first revision. Washington, DC: Department of State.

US State Department (2004) *Strategic Plan Fiscal Years 2004–2009: Security, Democracy, Prosperity*. Washington, DC: US Department of State and US Agency for International Development.

Varmus, Harold, R. Klausner, E. Zerhouni et al. (2003) 'Grand challenges in global health', *Science*, 302(5644), 398–9.

von Schirnding, Yasmin (2002) 'Health and sustainable development: can we rise to the challenge?', *Lancet*, 360, 632–7.

Vuori, Juha A. (2008) 'Illocutionary logic and strands of securitization: applying the theory of securitization to the study of non-democratic political orders', *European Journal of International Relations*, 14(1), 65–99.

Wald, Priscilla (2007) *Contagious: Cultures, Carriers and the Outbreak Narrative*. Durham, NC: Duke University Press.

Walker, R. B. J. (1993) *Inside/Outside: International Relations as Political Theory*. Cambridge: Cambridge University Press.

Walt, Stephen M. (1991) 'The renaissance of security studies', *International Studies Quarterly*, 35 (2), 211–239.

Waltz, Kenneth (1979) *Theory of International Politics*. Boston, MA: Addison-Wesley.

Wan, Xia, Shaojun Ma, Janet Hoek et al. (2011) 'Conflict of interest and FCTC implementation in China', *Tobacco Control*. Available at: http://tobaccocontrol.bmj.com/content/early/2011/06/14/tc.2010.041327.abstract

Weiner, Myron (1992–3) 'Security, stability, and international migration', *International Security*, 17(3), 91–126.

Wendt, Alexander (1992) 'Anarchy is what states make of it: the social construction of power politics', *International Organization*, 46(2), 391–425.

White, Caroline (2004) 'Global spending on health research still skewed towards wealthy nations', *British Medical Journal*, 329(7474), 1064. Available at: http://www.ncbi.nlm.nih.gov/pmc/articles/PMC526148.

White House [United States] (2002) *National Security Strategy of the United States*. Washington, DC: The White House.

White House (2009) *Statement by the President on [sic] Global Health Initiative*, 5 May. Available at: http://www.whitehouse.gov/the_press_office.

WHO [World Health Organization] (1946, amended 2006) *Constitution of the World Health Organization*. Available at: http://www.who.int/governance/eb/who_constitution_en.pdf.

WHO (1978) 'Declaration of Alma Ata on Primary Health Care'. Available at: http://www.who.int/hpr/NPH/docs/declaration_almaata.pdf.

WHO (1996) *The World Health Report 1996, Fighting Disease, Fostering Development*. Geneva: WHO.

WHO (2000) *Tobacco Company Strategies to Undermine Tobacco Control Activities at the World Health Organisation*, report of the Committee of Experts on Tobacco Industry Documents. Available at: http://www.who.int/tobacco/en/who_inquiry.pdf

WHO (2001) *Macroeconomics and Health: Investing in Health for Economic Development*, Report of the Commission on Macroeconomics and Health. Geneva: WHO.

WHO (2002) *Global Defense against the Infectious Disease Threat*. Geneva: WHO.

WHO (2007a) *The World Health Report 2007 – A Safer Future: Global Public Health Security in the 21st Century*. Geneva: WHO.

WHO (2007b) *Scientific Working Group on Life Science Research and Global Health Security: Report of First Meeting Geneva Switzerland, 16–18 October 2006*. Geneva: WHO.

WHO (2007c) 'World health day: high level debate tackled need for improved international health security'. Available at: http://www.who.int/world-health-day/previous/2007/activities.

WHO (2007d) 'Indonesia to resume sharing H5N1 avian influenza virus samples following a WHO meeting in Jakarta'. Available at: http://www.who.int/mediacentre/news/releases/2007/pr09/en/index.html.

WHO (2007e) 'The Right to Health', *Fact Sheet No. 323*. Geneva: WHO. Available at: http://www.who.int/mediacentre/factsheets/fs323/en/index.html

WHO (2008a) *Research Policy and Management of Risks in Life Sciences Research for Global Health Security: Report of the Meeting Bangkok, Thailand, 10–12 December 2007*. Geneva: WHO.

WHO (2008b) *Closing the gap in a generation: Health equity through action on the social determinants of health*, Commission on the Social Determinants of Health Final Report. Geneva: WHO.

WHO (2009) 'Availability, safety and quality of blood products', 125th Session of the Executive Board, EB125/5, 7 May. Available at: http://apps.who.int/gb/ebwha/pdf_files/EB125/B125_5-en.pdf.

WHO (2011) *Global Status Report on Non-communicable Diseases*. Geneva: WHO.

WHO (2012) 'HINARI Access to Research in Health Programme'. Available at: http://www.who.int/hinari/en/

WHO (no date) 'WHO Global Information Sharing Network'. Available at: http://www.who.int/csr/disease/influenza/surveillance/en/index.html.

WHO Europe (2007) *Towards Health Security*. Copenhagen: WHO Regional Office for Europe.

Wight, Martin (1979) *Power Politics*, (ed.) H. Bull and C. Holbraad. London: Pelican.

Willis, Carla Y. and Charlotte Leighton (1995), 'Protecting the poor under cost recovery: the role of means testing', *Health Policy and Planning*, 10, 241–56.

Wilson, Kimanan, Barbara von Tigerstrom and Christopher McDougall (2008) 'Protecting global health security through the International Health

Regulations: requirements and challenges', *Canadian Medical Association Journal*, 179(1), 44–8.

Wolinsky, Howard (2007) 'Bioethics goes global', *EMBO Reports*, 8(6), 534–6.

Woods, Ngaire (2001) 'International political economy in an age of globalization'. In J. Baylis and S. Smith (eds.) *The Globalization of World Politics*, 2nd edn. Oxford: Oxford University Press.

Woodward David, Nick Drager, Robert Beaglehole and Debra Lipson (2001) 'Globalization and health: A framework for analysis and action', *Bulletin of the World Health Organization*, 79, 875–81.

World Bank (1993) *World Development Report: Investing in Health*. Washington, DC: IBRD.

World Bank (2006) *About DCCP*. Available at: http://www.dcp2.org/page/main/About.html.

World Bank (2007) *Healthy Development: The World Bank Strategy for Health, Nutrition and Population Results*. Washington, DC: World Bank.

World Economic Forum/Harvard School of Public Health (2011) *The Global Economic Burden from Non-Communicable Diseases*, Geneva. Available at: http://www3.weforum.org/docs/WEF_Harvard_HE_GlobalEconomicBurdenNonCommunicableDiseases_2011.pdf.

World Medical Association [WMA] (2006) *Declaration of Geneva*. Available at: http://www.wma.net/en/30publications/10policies/g1/.

Youde, Jeremy (2010a) 'China's health diplomacy in Africa', *China: An International Journal*, 8(1), 151–63.

Youde, Jeremy (2010b) 'The relationship between foreign aid, HIV and government health spending', *Health Policy and Planning*, 25(6), 523–8.

Yuk-Ping, Catherine Lo and Nicholas Thomas (2010) 'How is health a security issue? Politics, responses and issues', *Health Policy and Planning*, 25(6), 447–53.

Zimmet, Paul Z. (2000) 'Globalization, coca-colonization and the chronic disease epidemic: Can the Doomsday scenario be averted?', *Journal of Internal Medicine*, 247(3), 301–10.

Index